D1188440

The Medicine of History
From Paracelsus to Freud

The Medicine of History
From Paracelsus to Freud

Harold L. Klawans, M.D.

Associate Chairman
Department of Neurological Sciences
Rush-Presbyterian-St. Luke's Medical Center
and
Professor
Departments of Neurological Sciences and Pharmacology
Rush University
Chicago, Illinois

Raven Press ■ New York

Raven Press, 1140 Avenue of the Americas, New York, New York 10036

Made in the United States of America

Library of Congress Cataloging in Publication Data

Klawans, Harold L.
    The medicine of history from Paracelsus
to Freud.

        Includes bibliographies.
        1. Neurology—Anecdotes, facetiae, satire,
etc.   2. Medicine—Anecdotes, facetiae, satire,
etc.   I. Title.   [DNLM: 1. Famous persons.
2. Neurology—History.   WL 11.1 K63m]
RC343.K5   616.8′09   82–489
ISBN 0–89004–684–0   AACR2

To my late father, Harold L. Klawans, who taught me how to look at many things.

To the late Clark Hopkins who taught me to see clearly what I was looking at.

To my father-in-law, Irving Barkan, who taught me the meaning of my own heritage.

To my children, Deborah, Rebecca, and Jonathan, who taught me the joy of learning this heritage.

Preface

All things considered, I suppose my late father is primarily responsible for this book. When I was growing up, he taught me to pursue each interest by reading about it exhaustively. In this way, I acquired a library about dinosaurs, ancient coins, and baseball. When I was a junior medical student and I decided to become a neurologist, I asked my teacher, Dr. John S. Garvin, what books I should buy. He told me to start with Walsh's *Clinical Neuro-Ophthalmology*. This was then a one volume, single author text that cost what was then an enormous amount: $28.50. I did as he advised and actually read most (but not all) of it. On that same visit to Login Brothers Medical Book Store, the same store where my father had purchased his medical books some 40 years earlier, I also acquired a copy of Webb Haymaker's "Founders of Neurology." This cost $7.50 as I recall and I read it from cover to cover. By this one act, I combined my vocation and my avocation. The history of neurology became part of my lifelong love affair with history. This volume is the result of this love affair. It has had a very long gestation period. Ever since I began to teach neurology, I have used vignettes from its history as part of my repertoire and have always found that imparting such tidbits within the context of teaching rounds not only made teaching more fun for me, but also a more meaningful and better remembered teaching experience for most of the students and residents. Over the years I collected more and more of these stories, and some of them have even come to have a life of their own.

In this book I have put together some of my favorite stories which I am sure many residents and students who made rounds with me will remember. I have also included others which are new since they never seemed to fit into the format of bedside teaching.

Much of the material presented here is not entirely original. History cannot be. I have included a "Note" at the end of each chapter listing the major relevant sources. A number of books must be recommended to anyone with a sincere interest in the history of neurology. These are:

1. Webb Haymaker's *Founders of Neurology*, now in a newer edition edited by Webb Haymaker and Francis Schillers.
2. Lawrence McHenry Jr.'s *Garrison's History of Neurology*.
3. Ralph Major's *History of Medicine* (my favorite short introduction to the history of medicine).

S. A. K. Wilson's *Neurology* has wonderful historical introductions to each disease, and the historical reviews of most classic neurologic disorders in the *Handbook of Clinical Neurology*, edited by Pierre Vinken and George Bruyn, are often unexpected treasures.

Harold L. Klawans

Contents

The Acromegaly of Maximinus

It is easier to conceive than describe the universal joy of the Roman world on the fall of the tyrant.

Edward Gibbon, *The Decline and Fall of the Roman Empire.*

The Acromegaly of Maximinus

For hundreds of years, collectors of Roman coins have been aware of the distinctive, if not peculiar, profile of Maximinus I, emperor of Rome from 235 to 238 C. E. (Fig.1). The coin portraiture of this emperor clearly illustrates his heavy features, prominent supraorbital ridge, and markedly protruding lower jaw, or prognathism. These features, taken together, are highly suggestive, if not truly pathognomonic, of a clinical diagnosis of acromegaly. The term *acromegaly* comes from two Greek words: *akron*, which means extremity or extreme, and *megale*, which means great. It is a descriptive term that has been applied to the well-known clinical disorder characterized by enlargement of the extremities, especially the hands and the feet, as well as the nose and jaw. Such a diagnosis not only would explain the peculiar facial features of Maximinus but also might shed some light on other aspects of his life.

Maximinus was from one of the semibarbarous tribes of the interior of Thrace, a Roman province that comprised much of modern Yugoslavia and Bulgaria. He was born in Thrace about 173 C. E. of an obscure family, the son of Micca, a Goth, and of Ababa, an Alanian.[1] Maximinus was not a Roman citizen by descent, because neither of his parents was a Roman citizen, nor by place of birth, because Thracians at that time were not automatically granted Roman citizenship. Ancient sources indicate that he must have obtained his citizenship while in the army, perhaps for service in the field under the governor of Dacia. The major events of his military career and his brief reign as emperor are well known. He attracted the notice of Emperor Septimius Severus (Fig.2) (193–211 C. E.) because of his extraordinary

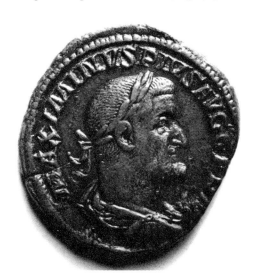

FIG. 1. Sestertius of Maximinus. MAXIMINUS PIVS AVG GERM. AVG: abbreviation for Augustus, which was the most distinctive title of the emperor. GERM: abbreviation for Germanicus, an honorary title given in reference to victories over German tribes. Often this title was also hereditary.

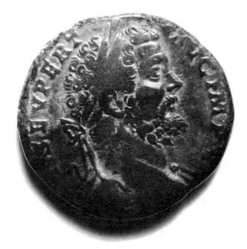

FIG. 2. Sestertius of Septimius Severus. SEV PERT AVG IMP V. SEV: abbreviation for Severus. PERT: abbreviation for Pertinax, predecessor of Septimius Severus as emperor. IMP: abbreviation for Imperator, a title of acclamation for victories of the emperor or his subordinates.

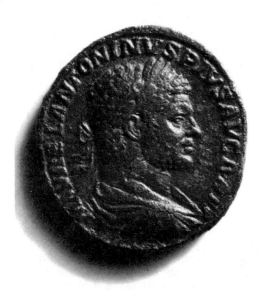

FIG. 3. Sestertius of Caracalla. M AVREL ANTONINUS PIUS AVG GERM.

size and strength, and he was given a military commission. During the reigns of Severus and his son Caracalla (Fig. 3) (211–217 C. E.), Maximinus attained the rank of centurion "with the favor and esteem of both those princes the former of whom was an excellent judge of merit."[2] Septimius Severus was a soldier of outstanding ability who was proclaimed emperor by his troops in 193 C. E. He reigned for 18 years and did much to strengthen the empire. At his death (211 C. E.) he left the empire to his two sons Caracalla and Geta (Fig. 4). After only 1 year Caracalla arranged for the assassination of Geta. Caracalla's reign was marked by

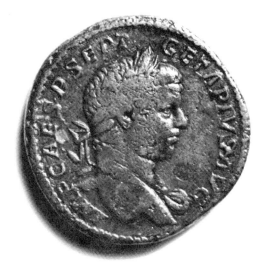

FIG. 4. Sestertius of Geta. IMP CAES P SEPT GETA PIUS AVG. CAES: abbreviation for Caesar, until adopted by all emperors and given to heirs to the throne.

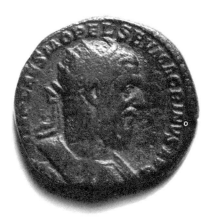

FIG. 5. As of Macrinus. IMP CAES M OPEL SEV MACRINUS AVG.

increasing cruelty and extravagance. In 217 C.E. he was murdered on the orders of the praetorian prefect Macrinus (Fig. 5), who was subsequently proclaimed emperor. Following the murder of Caracalla, Maximinus apparently left the army. Gibbon, basing his conclusions on *Scriptores Historia Augustae*,[1] explained Maximinus's resignation of his commission in these words: "Gratitude forbade Maximinus to serve under [Macrinus] the assassin of Caracalla."

Macrinus reigned for only 1 year. Although initially he was popular because he had disposed of the widely hated Caracalla, his popularity was short-lived. This change occurred primarily because of the unfavorable terms of the peace treaty he signed with Rome's archenemy, the Parthians. An open revolt of the Roman army in Syria resulted in the murder of Macrinus, with Elagabalus being proclaimed emperor (Fig. 6). Elagabalus was only 13 years old when he became emperor. His initial popularity with the army was quickly dissipated by 4 years of religious fanaticism, cruelty, bloodshed, and excesses of every description, and he was soon replaced on the throne by another youngster, his cousin Severus Alexander (Fig. 7). Gibbon also understood Maximinus's failure to serve under Elagabalus: "Honor taught him [Maximinus] to decline the effeminate insults of Elagabalus."

In 222 C. E., under Emperor Severus Alexander, Maximinus returned to military service.

> On the accession of Alexander he returned to court, and was placed by that prince in a station useful to the service and honourable to himself. The fourth

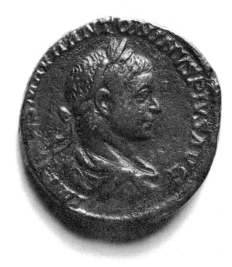

FIG. 6. Sestertius of Elagabalus. IMP CAES M AVG ANTONINUS PIUS AVG.

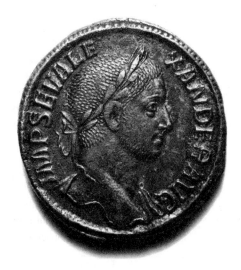

FIG. 7. Sestertius of Severus Alexander. IMP SEV ALEXANDER AVG.

legion, to which he was appointed tribune, soon became, under his care, the best disciplined of the whole army. With the general applause of the soldiers, who bestowed on their favourite hero the names of Ajax and Hercules, he was successively promoted to the first military command.[2]

It is believed that had Maximinus not still retained much of his savage origin, the emperor might have given his own sister in marriage to Maximus, the son of Maximinus.

The reign of Severus Alexander lasted only 13 years (222–235). This effeminate Syrian youth, who was under the thumb of his strong-willed mother Julia Mamaea, became increasingly unpopular with the army. In 235 C. E. the popular and well-loved Maximinus was proclaimed emperor by the army, and Severus Alexander was killed. Writing 1,500 years after the fact, Gibbon attributed to Maximinus a major role in engineering the coup, citing a variety of motives, including avarice and ambition:

> Instead of securing his fidelity, these favours served only to inflame the ambition of the Thracian peasant, who deemed his fortune inadequate to his merit, as long as he was constrained to acknowledge a superior. Though a stranger to real wisdom, he was not devoid of a selfish cunning, which showed him that the emperor had lost the affection of the army, and taught him to improve their discontent to his own advantage. It is easy for faction and calumny to shed their poison on the administration of the best of princes, and to accuse even their virtues, by artfully confounding them with those vices to which they bear the nearest affinity. The troops listened with pleasure to the emissaries of Maximin. They blushed at their ignominious patience, which, during thirteen years, had supported the vexatious discipline imposed by an effeminate Syrian, the timid slave of his mother and of the senate. It was time, they cried, to cast away that useless phantom of the civil power, and to elect for their prince and general a real soldier, educated in camps, exercised in war, who would assert the glory, and distribute among his companions the treasures of the empire. A great army was at that time assembled on the banks of the Rhine, under the command of the emperor himself, who, almost immediately after his return from the Persian war, had been obliged to march against the barbarians of Germany. The important care of training and reviewing the new levies was intrusted to Maximin. One day (A.D. 235, March 19), as he entered the field of exercise, the troops, either from a sudden impulse or a formed conspiracy, saluted him emperor, silenced by their loud acclamations his obstinate refusal, and hastened to consummate their rebellion by the murder of Alexander Severus.

TABLE 1. *Roman emperors during the career of Maximinus I*

Septimius Severus (Fig. 2)	193–211 C.E.
Caracalla (Fig. 3), son of Septimius Severus	211–217 C.E.
Geta (Fig. 4), son of Septimius Severus, murdered by Caracalla	211–212 C.E.
Macrinus (Fig. 5)	217–218 C.E.
Elagabalus (Fig. 6)	218–222 C.E.
Severus Alexander (Fig. 7)	222–235 C.E.
Maximinus (Figs. 1 and 8)	235–238 C.E.

Within 3 years of his accession the once-popular hero was considered to be a tyrant comparable to Caligula or Nero. According to all ancient sources, he was more of a monster than Caracalla. His cruelty was unbounded and was said to be exceeded only by his suspicious nature. Gibbon accused this once-honorable man of murdering many of his benefactors, leaving an indelible history of his baseness and ingratitude.

> The dark and sanguinary soul of the tyrant was open to every suspicion against those among his subjects who were the most distinguished by their birth or merit. Whenever he was alarmed with the sound of treason, his cruelty was unbounded and unrelenting. A conspiracy against his life was either discovered or imagined, and Magnus, a consular senator, was named as the principal author of it. Without a witness, without a trial, and without an opportunity of defence, Magnus with four thousand of his supposed accomplices, was put to death. Italy and the whole empire were infested with innumerable spies and informers. On the slightest accusation, the first of the Roman nobles who had governed provinces, commanded armies, and been adorned with the consular and triumphal ornaments, were chained on the public carriages, and hurried away to the emperor's presence. Confiscation, exile, or simple death, were esteemed uncommon instances of his lenity. Some of the unfortunate sufferers he ordered to be sewed up in the hides of slaughtered animals, others to be exposed to wild beasts, others again to be beated to death with clubs. During the three years of his reign, he disdained to visit either Rome or Italy. His camp, occasionally removed from the banks of the Rhine to those of the Danube, was the seat of his stern despotism, which trampled on every principle of law and justice, and was supported by the avowed power of the sword. No man of noble birth, elegant accomplishments, or knowledge of civil business, was suffered near his person; and the court of a Roman emperor revived the idea of those ancient chiefs of slaves and gladiators, whose savage power had left a deep impression of terror and detestation.

In the end, Maximinus (Fig. 8) and his son and heir Maximus (Fig. 9) were killed by the army.

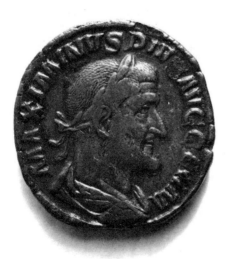

FIG. 8. Sestertius of Maximinus. MAX-MAXIMINUS PIUS AVG GERM.

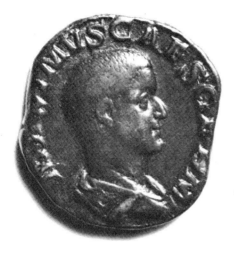

FIG. 9. Sestertius of Maximus.
MAXIMUS CAES GERM.

The distinctive features of the life of Maximinus include the following:

1. His prodigious size and strength;
2. An early record of honor, gratitude, and personal loyalty, and the ability to stimulate the love and loyalty of the army;
3. A later record of unbridled ambition, cruelty, and paranoid behavior that produced hatred and disloyalty among the same troops who only a few years earlier proclaimed him emperor.

At first glance there appears to be no obvious way to explain this personality change other than to attribute to Maximinus covert motives such as unbridled ambition and contempt for others that eventually became manifest. However, it is quite likely that a hormonally active pituitary tumor could, in part, account for all three of these features, especially in regard to understanding the abrupt change in his behavior.

The clinical syndrome of acromegaly was first described in 1886 by Pierre Marie (1853–1940). Marie is generally considered to have been the most able of Charcot's many students. His initial paper on acromegaly characterized the clinical manifestations of the disease and described its relationship to a tumor of the pituitary gland. It is now known that it is excessive production of growth hormone by the pituitary tumor that results in the extraordinary overgrowth of bone and the connective tissue of the skin and subcutaneous tissues. If the disorder sets in before the age at which the growth centers of the long bones of the arms and legs become joined, the bones grow enormously in all their dimensions, and the result is gigantism. But if the disorder begins after these growth centers have united, the overgrowth is confined to the ends of the bones, producing acromegaly. If the tumor begins before closure of the growth centers and continues its active production afterward the patient manifests both gigantism and acromegaly. This combination of pituitary gigantism and acromegaly was first described by another of Charcot's students, Henri Meige. Maximinus appears to have manifested both aspects of excessive growth hormone production.

Historical sources all agree that Maximinus was a giant, with reports of his height varying from 7 feet 2 inches to 8 feet 6 inches. As late as 1961, when the average height was certainly greater than it had been in the second and third centuries, it was generally taught that among Caucasians a body height in excess of 7 feet is almost always indicative of a pituitary tumor that is secreting growth hormone. This must also have been true 1,700 years ago.

The reports of Maximinus's height are accompanied by tales of his extraordinary, if not prodigious, strength. Although acromegaly usually is associated with weakness, there have been numerous reports of patients who were unusually strong early in the course of the disease and later gradually became weaker. In fact, Pierre Marie reported one such patient in his original paper.

Thus it is important to note that although Maximinus was reported to have exceptional strength, the descriptions of this strength derive from the period prior to his resignation from the army (217 C. E.) and mostly have to do with his initial meeting with Septimius Severus around the year 206. Borrowing directly from ancient sources, Gibbon retold these stories as follows:

> The Emperor Severus, returning from an eastern expedition, halted in Thrace, to celebrate, with military games, the birthday of his younger son, Geta [Fig. 4]. The country flocked in crowds to behold their sovereign, and a young barbarian of gigantic stature earnestly solicited, in his rude dialect, that he might be allowed to contend for the prize of wrestling. As the pride of discipline would have been disgraced in the overthrow of a Roman soldier by a Thracian peasant, he was matched with the stoutest followers of the camp, sixteen of whom he successively laid on the ground. His victory was rewarded by some trifling gifts, and a permission to enlist in the troops. The next day, the happy barbarian was distinguished above a crowd of recruits, dancing and exulting after the fashion of his country. As soon as he perceived that he had attracted the emperor's notice, he instantly ran up to his horse, and followed on foot, without the least appearance of fatigue, in a long and rapid career. "Thracian," said Severus, with astonishment, "art thou disposed to wrestle after thy race?" "Most willingly, Sir," replied the unwearied youth, and, almost in a breath, overthrew seven of the strongest soldiers in the army. A gold collar was the prize of his matchless vigour and activity, and he was immediately appointed to serve in the Horse-guards who always attended on the person of the sovereign.

There are no reports in any available ancient sources of extraordinary physical feats when Maximinus resumed his career under Severus Alexander (222 C. E.). All reports after this date deal with his administrative ability.

The manifestations of acromegaly are quite characteristic. There is progressive enlargement of the bones and soft parts that is most marked in the hands and feet, resulting, for instance, in broad, thick "gingerbread hands." In this regard it is particularly interesting to note that Maximinus's thumb was reported to be so thick that he used his wife's bracelet for a ring.[1] Such extreme thickness of the fingers and thumb is characteristic of acromegaly. Acromegaly also has characteristic effects on the skull and face. The skull becomes enlarged and thickened, and all its bony ridges are exaggerated; the margins of the orbits, including the supraorbital ridge, the cheekbones, the external occipital protuberance, and, most striking of all, the lower jaw, become enlarged. The mandible begins to jut out significantly, resulting in prognathism.

The coin portraiture of Maximinus (Figs. 1 and 8) demonstrates most of these features:

1. Marked prognathism
2. Marked supraorbital ridges
3. Overall gross features

It is of interest in regard to his physical features that he was often compared to Ajax, Achilles, and Hercules, but never to Adonis.[1] Herodian succinctly described Maximinus as "a man of frightening appearance and colossal size," a portrait that is consistent with combined gigantism and acromegaly.

According to the *Scriptores Historia Augustae*,[1] in a single day Maximinus could drink an amphora (about 7 gallons) of wine and eat 30 or 40 pounds of meat. Such degrees of thirst (polydipsia) and hunger (polyphagia), although undoubtedly exaggerated by this anonymous but wretched biographer, are far beyond the appetites attributed to other ancient heroes of noted strength and size. Polydipsia and polyphagia are, of course, two of the three cardinal symptoms of diabetes mellitus. The third is polyuria (excessive urination), which must occur in anyone who consumes anywhere near 7 gallons of fluid per day. Approximately 20% to 40% of acromegalics develop diabetes mellitus for one of two reasons: blockade of the action of insulin in the various tissues of the body; or exhaustion of those cells in the pancreas that manufacture insulin. It is quite possible that the increased consumption of both food and liquid attributed to Maximinus could have resulted from acromegaly-induced diabetes mellitus. Again the coin portraiture is of some help, because Maximinus's prodigious intake of food clearly was not associated with any evidence of obesity. This, of course, is most consistent with acromegaly-induced diabetes, in which increased appetite and food consumption result in no weight gain.

Thus far, the only aspects of the life of Maximinus that we have attributed to his pituitary tumor are those that were direct results of the growth hormone produced by the tumor. Such tumors can also produce symptoms by a second mechanism. The progressive slow growth of this tumor can cause pressure on neighboring structures, including the base of the brain, especially the hypothalamus, which lies directly over the pituitary. It is quite possible that extension of the tumor to involve the hypothalamus could help explain other aspects of Maximinus's career.

It is difficult to understand how this beloved and honorable man whose gratitude and loyalty to Severus forced him to resign from the army in 217 C. E., and who under Severus Alexander discharged his trust conscientiously, earning great popularity among his troops,[3] could a few years later become an ingrate, a despot of unbridled ambition.[2] It is difficult to imagine such degrees of ambition and cruelty in a man who once gave up his career out of a sense of loyalty and honor.

Whether or not Maximinus staged the coup that made him emperor, his troops clearly were pleased to proclaim their popular leader emperor. His troops loved Maximinus, despite the fact that he had made them the best disciplined legion in the entire army. Soldiers rarely love disciplinarians unless they are fair. But only 3 years later he was slain in his tent by a party of praetorian guards acting on orders of the Senate. This murder ended a 3-year reign that had been characterized by destructive rages, paranoid behavior, and cruel tyranny.

> Such was the deserved fate of the brutal savage, destitute, as he has generally been represented, of every sentiment that distinguishes a civilized, or even a human being. The body was suited to the soul. The stature of Maximin exceeded the measure of eight feet, and circumstances almost incredible are related of his match-less strength and appetite. Had he lived in a less enlightened age, tradition and poetry might well have described him as one of those monstrous giants, whose supernatural power constantly exerted for the destruction of mankind. It is easier to conceive than describe the universal joy of the Roman world on the fall of the tyrant.[2]

The monstrous change in Maximinus is difficult to understand on purely psychiatric grounds, but such changes in behavior have been described in patients with tumors involving the hypothalamus. Such patients can manifest increased emotional excitability, even building up to severe rage attacks, and aggressive behavior precipitated by paranoid ideation has been described as a characteristic sign of a tumor involving the hypothalamus. These patients can react to insignificant events with excessive states of excitement, and they are capable of indiscriminant attacks against anyone who happens to be present. Some of these patients have described this condition as a feeling of rage building up in spite of their efforts to control it, until it conquers their thoughts and leaves them no choice but to let it freely run its course. Other patients with this condition appear to wait in a state of tension for the first opportunity to release their accumulated aggressiveness.

It is tempting to speculate that Maximinus's pituitary tumor began to expand out of the sella turcica and slowly impinge on the hypothalamus. This would account for the vicious paranoid behavior that marked his cruel reign and led to his final destruction.

Absolute diagnosis, of course, would require an examination of the skeletal remains of Maximinus, but this will never be possible, because there is no chance that his body will ever be found. After Maximinus and his son were murdered, "their bodies were thrown out for anyone to desecrate and trample on before being left to be torn to pieces by dogs and birds."[3] The heads of Maximinus and his son were then sent to Rome and further desecrated before being thrown into the Tiber. Because his skull has been lost forever, there is no hope for pathological proof of the hypothesis that Maximinus represented the first recorded instance of acromegaly.

NOTES

The historical data presented here were for the most part derived from three sources:

1. *Scriptores Historia Augustae*, translated by D. Magie (Cambridge: Harvard University Press, 1968). This is a collection of biographies of Roman emperors, claimants to the throne, presumptive heirs, and colleagues from the time of Hadrian (117 C.E.) to Numerianus (284 C.E.). It was apparently compiled by six different anonymous authors between the years 285 and 335. The credibility and value of the individual biographies have been much debated.

2. Gibbon, E., *The Decline and Fall of the Roman Empire*.

3. Herodian, *History*, translated by C. R. Wittaker (Cambridge: Harvard University Press, 1969). The *History* of Herodian covers a period of the Roman Empire from the death of Emperor Marcus Aurelius (180 C.E.) to the accession of Gordian III (238 C.E.) just following the death of Maximinus. Most other sources for this period have been lost, so that Herodian's *History* is the only contemporary history of this era that has survived intact.

All coins illustrated here are from the collection of the author and were photographed by Harlan J. Berk, Ltd. The rendering of the coin inscriptions was done according to Klawans, Z. H., *Reading and Dating Roman Imperial Coins* (Racine, Wisc.: Western Publishing, 1977).

ADDENDUM: JOHN HUNTER'S GIANT

Nothing in nature stands alone; every art and science has a relation to some other art or science, and it requires a knowledge of these others, as far as this connexion takes place, to enable us to become perfect in that which engages our particular attention.

John Hunter

Mr. Hunter is the glory of England in this century. In vigour and originality of genius, in comprehension and depth of thought, in unwearied industry, he has been surpassed by none. He was one of the men who give a character to the age in which they live—whose names are associated with the great eras of science—and who do honour to the country which produced them.

William Lawrence

The notion that the diagnosis of combined acromegaly-gigantism in Maximinus could be substantiated if only we could find his skull is entirely reasonable. A similar diagnosis was made by the godfather of all pituitary tumors, Harvey Cushing, who examined the skull of John Hunter's giant only 150 years after the giant's death.

John Hunter (1728–1793) is generally considered to have been one of the greatest surgeons in the history of the United Kingdom, and he has often been referred to as the founder of scientific surgery. As one of his contemporary surgeons wrote of him, "He alone made us gentlemen." His numerous papers and publications did much to give the field of surgery a scientific outlook, but much of his time and energy was spent in amassing his once-famous collection.

This collection, which was not peculiar for its time, strikes us today as such. It was as much a menagerie as a scientific display of anatomical dissections. Additions to his collection often were sought after specifically because of their strangeness or grotesqueness. During his life, Hunter acquired and kept a whole host of live specimens, including leopards, snakes, buffaloes, bats, jackals, zebras, and an ostrich. Today, when many English estates have been turned into wildlife preserves as tourist attractions, one might not be surprised to find such a variety of animals in a country mansion. But Hunter's home was the first such preserve, and his motive was not monetary gain but an insatiable eclectic curiosity. His dead specimens included a famous racehorse and a greyhound that had belonged to a man of distinguished rank. The most famous skeletons were that of the great bone whale and that of the Irish giant named Bryrne or O'Brien. In classic Hunter style, the latter, which measured some 7 feet 6.5 inches, was displayed beside the skeleton of a Sicilian dwarf (1 foot 8 inches).

Hunter's zeal as a collector knew no bounds. From the time he first heard about the Irish giant Hunter coveted his remains. When the giant fell sick, Hunter knew his opportunity was near, and he spared neither time nor money. He was absolutely determined to have O'Brien's skeleton in his collection. As the giant was nearing death, Hunter had one of his assistants named Howisen keep a 24-hour watch over the dying man. The Irishman, however, knew something was afoot, and he was equally determined that his body would not be dissected and displayed. He arranged for his friends and an undertaker to keep a constant watch over his body from the time of death until a lead coffin could be built and his body sealed in it and buried at sea. Hunter offered the undertaker a bribe of £500, and soon after his death O'Brien's body became part of the Hunter collection.

In 1909 Harvey Cushing visited the Hunter collection, which had been purchased by the government on Hunter's death and had become the basis of the collection of the Royal College of Surgeons. Cushing examined the skull of Hunter's giant and found that the sella turcica was eroded and that this erosion had been caused by a pituitary tumor. Thus O'Brien's acromegaly-gigantism was due to a pituitary tumor, and the Irish giant, who died more than 100 years before Marie's original paper, became the first proven case of pituitary acromegaly. The local inhabitants of the community where O'Brien had been born had a different interpretation. They attributed the giant's extraordinary size to a supernatural influence of the site of his conception, although it is unclear how the specific site was known to them.

The Norwegian Explorer

Some get a kick from cocaine.
I'm sure that if
I took even one sniff,
it would bore me terrifically too.

Cole Porter, "I Get a Kick Out of You" from *Anything Goes*, 1934

The Norwegian Explorer

On May 4, 1891, Mr. Sherlock Holmes, the first and most renowned of the world's consulting detectives, disappeared, apparently having fallen into the chasm that is Reichenbach Falls in a final struggle to the death with Moriarty, the infamous Napoleon of crime. In *The Final Problem*, Dr. John H. Watson, who had hurried back to the top of the falls only to find a farewell note from Holmes, described the scene in these words:

> A few words may suffice to tell the little that remains. An examination by experts leaves little doubt that a personal contest between the two men ended, as it could hardly fail to end in such a situation, in their reeling over, locked in each other's arms. Any attempt at recovering the bodies was absolutely hopeless, and there, deep down in that dreadful cauldron of swirling water and seething foam, will lie for all time the most dangerous criminal and the foremost champion of the law of their generation. . . . As to the gang, it will be within the memory of the public how completely the evidence which Holmes had accumulated exposed their organization, and how heavily the hand of the dead man weighed on them.

Almost 3 years later, on April 5, 1894, Holmes once again appeared in London. Where had he been during those 3 years he had been presumed dead, and why had he remained away so long? According to Holmes, he stayed underground to avoid the dangerous remnants of Moriarty's organization.

Holmes returned to 221B Baker Street to dispose of Colonel Sebastian Moran, the last surviving henchman of Moriarty (see *The Adventure of the Empty House*). He offered Watson the following explanation of his whereabouts during the previous 3 years:

> I travelled for two years in Tibet, therefore, and amused myself by visiting Lhassa and spending some days with the head Llama. You may have read of the remarkable explorations of a Norwegian named Sigerson, but I am sure that it never occurred to you that you were receiving news of your friend. I then passed through Persia, looked in at Mecca, and paid a short but interesting visit to the Khalifa at Khartoum, the results of which I have communicated to the Foreign Office. Returning to France I spent some months in a research into the coal-tar derivatives, which I conducted in a laboratory at Montpelier, in the South of France. Having concluded this to my satisfaction, and learning that only one of my enemies was now left in London, I was about to return when my movements were hastened by the news of this remarkable Park Lane Mystery, which not only appealed to me by its own merits, but which seemed to offer some most peculiar personal opportunities.

Few, if any, scholars accept this obvious fabrication. Baring-Gould, one of the greatest of the Holmes biographers, has suggested that much of these three missing years during which he had been presumed dead were spent enjoying a liaison with Irene Adler in Montenegro. Irene Adler appears in only one adventure, *A Scandal in Bohemia*, but "to Sherlock Holmes she is always the woman. . . . In his eyes she eclipses and predominates the whole of her sex."

This information would certainly have astounded Watson, who always believed that all emotions, and love particularly, were abhorrent to Holmes's cold, precise, but admirably balanced mind. As living proof of this relationship, Baring-Gould has claimed that Nero Wolfe is the by-product of the illicit love affair between Holmes and Adler. Wolfe, whose adventures have been so ably recounted by Rex Stout, was born in Montenegro and does combine the tastes of Irene Adler, the logical mind of Sherlock Holmes, and the corpulent body of Holmes's brother, Mycroft Holmes.

Dr. David Musto, in a 1968 article in the *Journal of the American Medical Association*, offered an alternative solution. He proposed that for much of those 3 years Holmes was in Vienna, living in the home of Dr. Sigmund Freud and being treated by Freud for cocaine addiction. This same hypothesis was expanded by Nicholas Meyer in his novel *The Seven Percent Solution* and is now widely believed. Thus, we are asked to believe that Holmes, the possessor of an "admirably balanced mind," was a victim of cocaine addiction and that he traveled all the way to Vienna to be treated by a man who at that time was a rather obscure neurologist. This was supposed to have occurred a decade or more before psychoanalysis was born. At that time in his career, Freud's major claim to fame was having translated the lectures of Jean Charcot from French into German (Fig. 1), an endeavor that would hardly have made him well known in English-language countries. The cocaine-Freud hypothesis seems to raise more questions than it answers. Was Holmes really a cocaine addict? How could Holmes have heard of Freud? And, more precisely, how did Holmes know that Freud knew of the dangers of cocaine addiction and was actively trying to cure such patients when all of Freud's earlier German-language publications had proclaimed the wonders of cocaine and denied that cocaine itself had any addicting properties?

In order to understand the involvement of Holmes and Freud with cocaine, some understanding of the emergence and impact of cocaine on nineteenth-century Europe is necessary. Cocaine is a product of the Western Hemisphere. It is an alkaloid derived from two species of shrubs of the genus *Erythroxylon*. Bolivian coca (*E. coca*) is native to the Andes highland forests, although a closely related variety grows in the Amazon lowland basin. Colombian coca (*E. novogranatense*) grows in Colombia, Venezuela, and the desert coast of Peru. Coca, of course, should not be confused with the cocoa, or cacao, plant, the seeds of which are the source of chocolate.

By the time Europeans first reached South America, the use of coca, the source of cocaine, was already widespread and well established. Manco Cepac, the royal son of the Inca Sun God, was believed to have given coca directly to the Incas, and the Inca priests, in turn, had declared that coca was divine. In the Inca culture, coca was consumed by being chewed in a mixture called *cocada*. This preparation was made up of coca itself, an alkali that would act to release the alkaloid from the coca leaves, and some sort of binding material. The importance of coca in the pre-Colombian cultures is shown by the fact that the term *cocada* came to be used

Neue Vorlesungen

über die

Arthur R. Edwards-
Vienna 793-

Krankheiten des Nervensystems

insbesondere über Hysterie.

Von

J. M. CHARCOT.

Autorisirte deutsche Ausgabe

von

DR. SIGM. FREUD,

Docent für Nervenkrankheiten an der k. k. Universität in Wien.

Mit 59 Abbildungen.

LEIPZIG UND WIEN.
TOEPLITZ & DEUTICKE.
1886.

FIG. 1. Title page of the German edition of Charcot's *Diseases of the Nervous System*, translated by Sigmund Freud. (Courtesy Paul A. Nausieda, M. D.)

as a measure of distance (the distance a man could walk under the influence of cocaine) or time (40 minutes, or the duration of action of cocaine taken orally).

The first description of the peculiar effects of coca to reach Europe was written in the sixteenth century by Nicholas Monardes of Spain (Fig. 2), but the plant seems to have aroused little, if any, interest until the middle of the nineteenth century. Nicholas Monardes was born the year after Columbus first sailed toward his discovery of the New World. He died in 1588. He was educated at the University of Alcala des Henares, which during the sixteenth century was a major seat of learning in western Europe. Following graduation, he began the practice of medicine in his native city of Seville, but he maintained a scholarly interest in botany and especially the medicinal uses of plants from the New World that he was able to have sent to him in Seville. His book was written in 1569 and translated into English in 1577 by John Frampton. Despite its title, *Joyfull Newes Out of the Newe Founde*

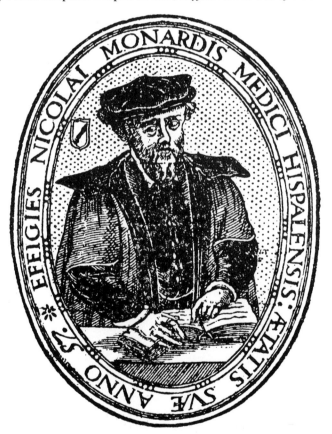

FIG. 2. Woodcut portrait of N. Monardes (1493–1588). (From *Dos Libros*. Seville: H. Diaz, 1569, courtesy of the Wellcome Trustees, Wellcome Institute for the History of Medicine, London, England.)

Worlde, this was not a paean in praise of cocaine but a serious compendium of a variety of New World plants and their effects. One of these, of course, was coca:

> I was desirous to see that hearbe so celebrated of the Indians, so many yeres past, which they do call the Coca, which they doe sow and till with muche care and diligence because they use it for their pleasures, which we will speake of.
>
> The use of it amongst the Indians is a thing generall, for many things, for when they travell by the waye, for neede and for their content when they are in their houses they use it in this forme. They take Cockles or Oysters, in theyr shelles and burne them and grinde them, after they are burned they remaine like Lime, very small ground: then they take the leaves of the Coca, and chewe them in theyr Mouthes, and as they chewe it, they mingle it with some of the pouder made of the shelles in such sorte, that they make it like a paste, taking less of the Pouder than of the herbe, and of this Paste they make certeyne small bawles round, and lay them to drie, & when they will use them, they take a little Ball in their mouth, and chewe it rowling it from one place to an other, procuring to conserve it all they can, and that being done, they take an other, and so they goe, using it al the time that they have need, which is when they travell by the waye, and especially if it be by ways where is no meate, nor plentie of water. For the use of these little Balles taketh the hunger and thirst from them: & they say that they receive substaunce thereby, as though they did eat meate. At other tymes they use them for their pleasure, although they labour not by the waye, and they use the Coca alone, chewing and tossing it in their mouths, from side to another, until there be no vertue remaining in it and then they take another.
>
> When they will make themselves drunke, and be out of judgement, they mingle with the Coca the leaves of the Tobaco, and chewe them altogether, and goe as it were out of their wittes, or as if they were drunke, which is a thing that dooth give them great contentment, to be in that sort. Surely it is a thing of great consideration, to see howe desirous the Indians are to be deprived of their wittes, and to bee without understanding, seeing that they use thus the Coca with the Tabaco, and al to this end . . .

Although Monardes must be given credit for publishing the first account of the divine plant of the Incas, he had no clear idea of its medicinal potentialities either for good or for evil.

Most European readers and potential users of herbs were much more interested in another plant he described: tobacco. Even the words of the Inca chronicler Garcilaso de la Vega, who wrote in 1609 that "coca satisfies the hungry, gives new strength to the weary and exhausted and makes the unhappy forget their sorrows," could not "turn on" seventeenth-century Europeans.

In 1859 the Italian physician Paola Montegazza published a report entitled *Sulle virtu igeniche e medicinali della coca*. It may be more than a coincidence that three other books destined to influence Western civilization were also published that same year: *Das Kapital*, *Uncle Tom's Cabin*, and *The Origin of Species*. This pamphlet was based on Montegazza's experiences during his travels among Peruvian Indians, and it proclaimed that coca was a wondrous new weapon against various diseases.

Unlike the little-noticed work of Monardes, Montegazza's report attracted a great deal of attention. The next year, Alfred Niemann, a Viennese biochemist, succeeded in purifying coca alkaloid, and he named it cocaine. The alkaloid had previously been partially isolated by Gaedicke and called exythroxylon. The first scientific reports were relatively unenthusiastic, but at that time the degree of quality control in the processing of coca leaves and coca extracts was poor at best.

Although the scientific community was slow to study cocaine, the public was quick to take up its use. In 1865, Vin Mariani, a preparation of wine and coca leaves, was placed on the market (Fig. 3). By 1890, a wide variety of cocaine nostrums were being sold, including cocaine cordials and even coca cigarettes. The foremost of these was Coca-Cola. The popular press carried many articles proclaiming the wonders of cocaine. Sherlock Holmes was a voracious reader of the popular press, and he must have been well aware of the alleged potentials of cocaine.

But was Holmes a cocaine addict? The answer is emphatically "Yes!" In *A Scandal in Bohemia* (probably late 1886), Watson tells us that Holmes, "who loathes every form of society with his whole Bohemian soul, remained in our lodgings in Baker Street, buried among his old books, and alternating from week to week between cocaine and ambition, the drowsiness of the drug, and the fierce energy of his own keen nature." Watson, who had seen little of Holmes because of his recent marriage, called on Holmes at their old lodgings and noted that Holmes had" risen out of his drug-created dreams and was hot upon the scent of some new problem."

The next year, in *The Man With the Twisted Lip*, Watson worries that Holmes's drug habits may be expanding. "I suppose, Watson," said he, "that you imagine that I have added opium smoking to cocaine injections, and all the other weaknesses on which you have favored me with your medical views." But no, Holmes was in the opium den in pursuit of an enemy. A few months later Watson repeated to Holmes his listing of Holmes's limits *(The Five Orange Pips)*:

> It was a singular document. Philosophy, astronomy, and politics were marked at zero, I remember. Botany variable, geology profound as regards to the mud-stains from any region within fifty miles of town, chemistry eccentric, anatomy unsystematic, sensational literature and crime records unique, violin-player, boxer, swordsman, lawyer, and self-poisoner by cocaine and tobacco. Those, I think, were the main points of my analysis.

The next year (1888) Watson reports the following: "Save for the occasional use of cocaine, he had no vices, and he only turned to the drug as a protest against the monotony of existence when cases were scanty and the papers uninteresting" *(The Yellow Face)*. The longest discussion of his cocaine habit appears in *The Sign of the Four* (1888).

> Sherlock Holmes took his bottle from the corner of the mantelpiece, and his hypodermic syringe from its neat morocco case. With his long, white, nervous fingers he adjusted the delicate needle and rolled back his left shirtcuff. For some little time his eyes rested thoughtfully upon the sinewy forearm and wrist, all dotted and scarred with innumerable puncture-marks. Finally, he thrust the sharp point home, pressed down the tiny piston, and sank back into the velvet-lined armchair with a long sigh of satisfaction.
>
> Three times a day for many months I had witnessed this performance, but custom had not reconciled my mind to it. . . .
>
> "Which is it to-day," I asked, "morphine or cocaine?"

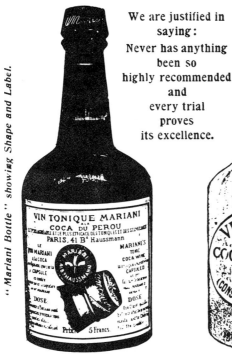

"*Mariani Bottle*" *showing Shape and Label.*

We are justified in
saying:
Never has anything
been so
highly recommended
and
every trial
proves
its excellence.

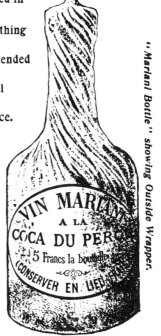

"*Mariani Bottle*" *showing Outside Wrapper.*

Size of Regular Bottle, half litre (about 17 ounces).

Never sold in bulk — to guard against substitution.

VIN MARIANI

Nourishes - Fortifies
Refreshes
Aids Digestion - Strengthens the System.

Unequaled as a tonic-stimulant for fatigued or
overworked Body and Brain.

Prevents Malaria, Influenza and Wasting Diseases.

We cannot aim to gain support for our preparation through cheapness; we give a uniform, effective and honest article, and respectfully ask personal testing of **Vin Mariani** strictly on its own merits. Thus the medical profession can judge whether **Vin Mariani** is deserving of the unequaled reputation it has earned throughout the world during more than 30 years.

Inferior, so-called Coca preparations (variable solutions of Cocaine and cheap wines) which have been proven worthless, even harmful in effect, bring into discredit and destroy confidence in a valuable drug.

We therefore particularly caution to specify always " VIN MARIANI,"
thus we can guarantee invariable satisfaction to physician and patient.

FIG. 3. Advertisement for a cocaine-containing nostrum. (Courtesy Yale Medical Library.)

He raised his eyes languidly from the old black-letter volume which he had opened.

"It is cocaine," he said, "a seven-per-cent solution. Would you care to try it?"

"No, indeed," I answered brusquely. "My constitution has not got over the Afghan campaign yet. I cannot afford to throw any extra strain upon it."

He smiled at my vehemence. "Perhaps you are right, Watson," he said. "I suppose that its influence is physically a bad one. I find it, however, so transcendentally stimulating and clarifying to the mind that its secondary action is a matter of small moment. . . .

"My mind," he said, "rebels at stagnation. Give me problems, give me work, give me the most obtuse cryptogram, or the most intricate analysis, and I am in my own proper atmosphere. I can dispense then with artificial stimulants. But I abhor the dull routine of existence. I crave for mental exaltation."

It is abundantly clear that by 1891 Holmes was a confirmed cocaine addict. No reference to active cocaine abuse appears in any stories dated later than his return to London in 1894. In *The Adventure of the Missing Three-quarter*, which occurred in 1896, Watson remarks that Holmes has been weaned of his drug mania, but he still worries that a period of idleness could give rise to a rebirth of Holmes's craving for an artificial stimulus. The evidence strongly points not only to cocaine addiction on Holmes's part but also to an addiction that was cured at some time between 1891 and 1894.

By the 1880s, abuse of cocaine was widespread. However, Sigmund Freud's interest in cocaine was not because of its potential for abuse but because of the realistic possibility that cocaine could have therapeutic uses. How had Freud become aware of the potential medical uses of cocaine? The first published reports of medical use of coca and its alkaloid derivatives appeared in American medical periodicals. In 1876, writing in the quite prestigious *Boston Medical and Surgical Journal*, Dr. G. A. Stockwell described numerous possible therapeutic benefits from coca, provided, of course, that it was not used in excess. Stockwell proclaimed that coca eliminated fatigue without ever causing depression and that there was "no recoil" from the use of this agent. He concluded that "the moderate use of coca is not only wholesome but frequently beneficial." He believed that only alarmists could be worried about any possible habituation.

Four years later, several articles in the *Therapeutic Gazette* suggested that coca was a "new cure for the opium habit," whereby coca could be used by addicts in place of opium, and after it had replaced opium, the coca could be easily and safely withdrawn. This would leave the former addict free of addiction. First, Edward D. Huse suggested that erythroxylon coca could cure the opium habit, whereas W. H. Bentley and A. F. Stimmel, in separate articles, claimed that coca could cure both alcoholism and opium addiction. Dr. Bentley further claimed that coca could cure a variety of other chronic diseases ranging from dyspepsia to tuberculosis. Numerous other American reports were equally enthusiastic.

A great deal of information on the therapeutic uses of coca-cocaine had been published by the 1880s and thus was available to Freud, but why would he be particularly interested? Freud's interest in cocaine was specifically stimulated by these articles, because Freud himself was frantically searching for a cure for morphine addiction.

By 1883 Freud had become a close friend of Ernst Fleischl (1846–1891) (Fig. 4). This friendship had begun when they were studying together in Vienna. Fleischl had been a brilliant physiologist who apparently had developed a traumatic neuroma

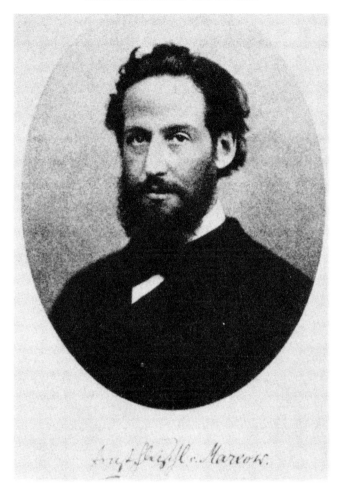

FIG. 4. Photograph of Ernst Fleischl von Marxow. (From Mary A. B. Brazier, *A History of the Electrical Activity of the Brain,* 1961, Pitman Medical Publishing Co., London, with permission.)

following a thumb amputation. It is said that he had turned to morphine for relief of his pain and had become a morphine addict. Whatever the exact circumstances of his acquiring the morphine habit, there is no question that he was addicted. Those who are skeptical may question the reason behind Fleischl's addiction. When persons of Fleischl's stature become drug addicts, their biographers and historians almost invariably find some socially acceptable basis for the addiction (e.g., the addiction of Eugene O'Neill's mother, which is always said to have a medical basis). Persons without biographers to defend them seem never to have such exogenous causes for their addictions. Freud, stimulated by what he had read in the American literature, wrote for and obtained a shipment of cocaine from Eli Merck in the hope of curing his friend and colleague.

After several months of administering cocaine to Fleischl, and also taking it himself, Freud wrote the first of his five articles on coca. This article, "Über Coca," was a glowing report that suggested seven therapeutic applications for coca:

1. To increase the physical capacity of the body for a given short period of time and to hold strength in reserve for wartime;
2. In digestive disorders of the stomach;
3. In cachexia;
4. To counteract the morphine withdrawal syndrome;
5. In asthma;
6. As a sexual stimulant, or aphrodisiac;
7. As a local anesthetic.

Freud did not claim to have discovered all of these uses himself. He clearly credited Bentley as having been the first to demonstrate the value of cocaine for the treatment of both morphine addiction and alcoholism. However, Freud did not merely repeat Bentley's original claims. He extended them and proclaimed that cocaine was so potent and specific in both morphine addiction and alcohol addiction that with its use alcohol asylums could soon be entirely eliminated.

So Freud knew and loved cocaine. He proclaimed its virtures early and often. His interest in cocaine was widely known. In print, Freud always maintained that cocaine was a wonder drug and by itself was not addicting. Why would Sherlock Holmes seek out Freud as the physician to treat addiction to a drug that Freud considered a wonder drug?

Unfortunately for both Freud and Fleischl, cocaine was no more successful as a cure for morphine addiction than was heroin, which also had originally been introduced for this purpose. Reports like the one that appeared in *The Lancet* on November 1, 1890, began to surface, suggesting that cocaine itself was addicitng (Fig. 5).

As the scientific and medical community became increasingly aware of the dangers of cocaine, Freud began to realize its limitations. Fleischl was far from being cured, and he soon became a pathetic example of cocaine addiction. By April 1885, Fleischl was injecting about 1 gram of cocaine each day, and Freud spent many long soul-searching nights at Fleischl's bedside. Fleischl died in 1891, the same year Holmes traveled to Vienna to come under Freud's care.

The professional career of Ernst Fleischl, who often signed his papers with his full name, Fleischl von Marxow, was also tainted by controversy. In 1890, Adolf Beck (Figs. 6 and 7), who was an assistant in the physiology department of the University of Jagiellianski in Krakau, Poland, published his thesis on alterations in the brain's steady state potentials due to sensory stimulation, and at the same time he described spontaneous electrical activity (brain waves). Beck apparently was unaware that both of these phenomena had previously been demonstrated by Caton, and he published a three-page abstract of his thesis in German in the "*Centralblatt für Physiologie*." Fleischl, then a professor of physiology at the University of Vienna, immediately sent a letter to the editor of the *Centralblatt*. In this letter he revealed that two sealed letters could be found in the archives of the University

THE LANCET.

LONDON: SATURDAY, NOVEMBER 1, 1890.

COCAINE CRAVING.

To the Editors of THE LANCET.

SIRS,—I have a patient who suffers from cocaine craving. I find it impossible to keep cocaine out of his reach. This habit has brought him into a very low state of health. Perhaps some of your readers might be able to give me some suggestion as to treatment. I have tried the usual remedies in vain. He suffers from great nervousness, sleeplessness, and has become very thin.—I am, Sirs, yours truly,

Oct. 28th, 1890. IRENE.

FIG. 5. An early testimony to the danger of cocaine.

of Vienna that would demonstrate that he, not Beck, had originally observed these phenomena. The letters were opened at a session of the Imperial Academy of Science on November 20, 1890. The first letter, dated November 7, 1883, entitled "Physiological discovery to be worked on further" and initialed E.F., did demonstrate that Fleischl had observed that sensory stimulation did produce potential shifts. He did not, on the other hand, clearly observe spontaneous potentials, but he nevertheless claimed priority for the discovery of brain potentials. Although the practice of depositing sealed envelopes containing scientific discoveries, rather than publishing the new information, seems strange at best, it was not unknown in the 1880s. However, the entire episode has a peculiar, if not paranoid-grandiose, flavor. This raises the question whether or not some of Fleischl's behavior could represent cocaine-induced psychosis, whether his claims were no more based on reality than Holmes's view of Moriarty. Because Fleischl von Marxow's depositing of the sealed envelope, as well as the work he described in it, occurred while he was being "cured" of his opium habit by taking injections of cocaine, this is more than just a vague possibility. Beck, like Fleischl, came to a tragic end. After a long and productive life he was murdered by the Nazis at the age of 79 for three capital crimes: He was a Jew. He was a Polish patriot. He was an intellectual.

Privately, then, Freud knew something of the dangers of cocaine and was attempting to treat cocaine addiction in at least one case. What was his public stance? Freud never publicly retracted his broad endorsement of cocaine. However, he did finally agree that it was not a cure for morphine addiction.

Freud's papers on cocaine caused controversy and even rebuke. The great Erlenmeyer carried out his own careful study of the use of cocaine in morphine

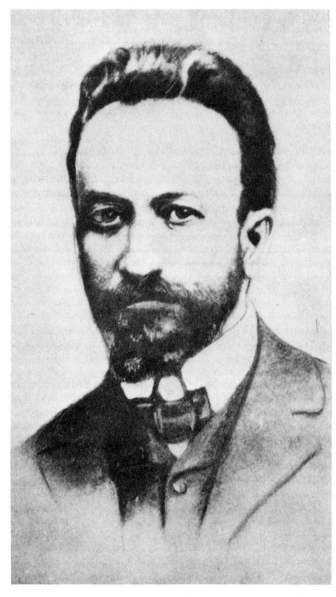

FIG. 6. Adolf Beck during the period of his doctoral work. (From Mary A. B. Brazier, *A History of the Electrical Activity of the Brain*, 1961, Pitman Medical Publishing Co., London, with permission.)

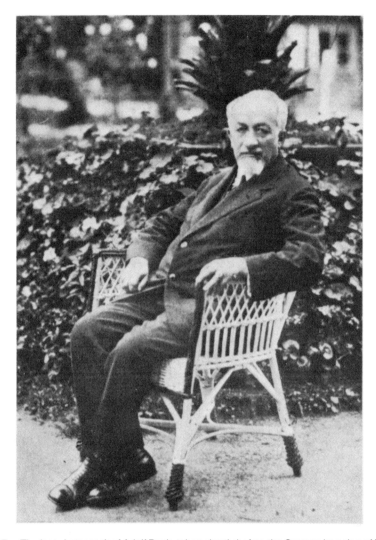

FIG. 7. The last photograph of Adolf Beck, taken shortly before the German invasion of Poland. (From Mary A. B. Brazier, *A History of the Electrical Activity of the Brain*, 1961, Pitman Medical Publishing Co., London, with permission.)

addiction and denounced its use. Further than just attacking cocaine, Erlenmeyer also denounced Freud for propagating what he called the "third scourge of mankind" (alcohol and morphine ranked as the first two). In this way Freud became the first scientist to be personally blamed for a major drug disaster. Freud himself never accepted Erlenmeyer's conclusions. He claimed that Erlenmeyer's work could not be compared to his, because Erlenmeyer gave his patients cocaine subcutaneously, whereas Freud had at least once suggested its oral use. However, as noted earlier, Fleischl, the one morphine addict whose cocaine therapy under Freud was well documented, injected cocaine. Nonetheless, Freud did withdraw his support for cocaine as a cure for morphine addiction. He did not do this because of recognition that cocaine itself was capable of causing addiction, but because he believed that the personalities of addicts were such that they transferred their tendency for addiction. He believed that such persons were so weak in willpower and so susceptible that cocaine merely replaced morphine. Freud still believed that cocaine itself was not addicting, stating that "cocaine has claimed no victim who has not previously been addicted to another drug." Freud's fifth and final paper on cocaine was published in 1887, only 3 years after his enthusiastic, if not proselytizing, article "Über Coca." In the following years he rarely, if ever, publicly discussed this cocaine interlude. In analytic terms, the entire adventure had resulted in a narcissistic injury that he consciously tried to suppress.

Given Freud's public stance, how would Sherlock Holmes or his medical amanuensis have known that Freud recognized the dangers of cocaine addiction and was actually treating patients for cocaine addiction. Nicholas Meyers would have us believe that Dr. Stamford, an obscure pathologist whose only claim to fame was that he originally introduced Watson and Holmes, knew of Freud's work. How Stamford, quietly pursuing pathology in the basement of St. Bartholomew's Hospital in London, would know of these unpublished interests of a Vienese neurologist is never explained. The only works of Freud that Stamford might have read had denied that cocaine was addicting.

Only someone who either knew Freud or had connections in Vienna who knew Freud would have known Freud's real feelings about cocaine. The fact that Irene Adler was a citizen of the Austro-Hungarian Empire raises the possibility that some member of her family in Vienna may have known Freud. One might think that her cousin, Alfred Adler, one of Freud's most distinguished students, would have been the missing link. Unfortunately, this cannot be the answer. Freud's experience with cocaine antedated his interest in psychoanalysis by many years, and Adler did not become his protégé until 10 years after Holmes returned to London.

David Musto has suggested that the note in *The Lancet* signed "Irene" (Fig. 5) was from Watson (using the name of "that woman," Irene Adler) and that an answer to this query may have supplied Watson with the needed answer. But the answer could have come only from someone who knew Freud closely, who knew his innermost feelings. Who could that have been?

As always, the best way to solve a problem involving Sherlock Holmes is to study the stories as told by John Watson, M. D., and recorded by Arthur Conan Doyle, M. D. In *The Adventure of the Empty House* Holmes himself supplies the answer: "You may have read of the remarkable explorations of a Norwegian named Sigerson, but I am sure that it never occurred to you that you were receiving news of your friend." The name Sigerson, the name chosen by Holmes to cover his missing 3 years, supplies the answer. Who, then, was this man Sigerson whose

LECTURES

MICHAEL REESE HOSPITAL

Dr. Bauga memorial

ON

THE DISEASES OF

THE NERVOUS SYSTEM.

DELIVERED AT LA SALPÊTRIÈRE

BY

J. M. CHARCOT,

PROFESSOR TO THE FACULTY OF MEDICINE OF PARIS; PHYSICIAN TO LA SALPÊTRIÈRE; MEMBER OF
THE ACADEMY OF MEDICINE, AND OF THE CLINICAL SOCIETY OF LONDON; PRESIDENT
OF THE ANATOMICAL SOCIETY, AND EX-VICE-PRESIDENT OF THE
BIOLOGICAL SOCIETY OF PARIS, ETC.

TRANSLATED FROM THE SECOND EDITION BY

GEORGE SIGERSON, M.D., M.Ch.,

LICENTIATE OF THE KING AND QUEEN'S COLLEGE OF PHYSICIANS; LECTURER ON BIOLOGY AND
EX-DEAN OF THE FACULTY OF SCIENCE, CATHOLIC UNIVERSITY OF IRELAND; FELLOW OF
THE LINNEAN SOCIETY OF LONDON; MEMBER OF THE SCIENTIFIC SOCIETY OF
BELGIUM, AND OF THE ROYAL IRISH ACADEMY, ETC.

WITH ILLUSTRATIONS.

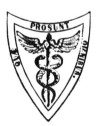

PHILADELPHIA:

HENRY C. LEA.

1879.

FIG. 8. Title page of the English edition of Charcot's *Diseases of the Nervous System*, translated by George Sigerson. (Courtesy Paul A. Nausieda, M. D.)

name Holmes relayed to us? He certainly was not a Norwegian explorer. He was a neurologist: George Sigerson, M. D. Sigerson was not just your average neurologist, but a man of great accomplishments and renown, as shown by his published list of honors:

> Licentiate of the King and Queen's College of Physicians of Ireland; Dean of the Faculty of Science, C. U. I., Member of the Royal Irish Academy: Fellow of the Linnean Society of London; Member of Council of Statistical Society, Dublin; Member of the Scientific Society of Brussels; Corresponding Member of the Clinical and Anthropological Societies of Paris, etc.

But was Sigerson in a position to know Freud's true feelings about cocaine and cocaine addiction?

Sigerson, like Freud, had attended Charcot's lectures at the Salpêtrière and was, like Freud, a student of the father of French neurology. Sigmund Freud had translated Charcot's lectures on the diseases of the nervous system into German (Fig. 1), and George Sigerson had translated these same lectures into English (Fig. 8). As with many other students who find themselves coming together to learn under the same master, a bond had been established between Freud and Sigerson. As a result of this bond, Sigerson was probably the only person in Great Britain in a position to know Freud's new position on cocaine. Therefore it must have been Sigerson who answered the plea signed "Irene" and was instrumental in introducing Freud and Holmes. The latter's assumption of the name Sigerson is his public expression of thanks to the physician who made it possible for him to spend some time with the head lama of psychoanalysis. Whether or not Holmes influenced Freud's future thinking, as suggested by Musto, Freud obviously influenced Holmes's, and for that we must all be thankful.

It is of interest that several generations of Sherlock Holmes scholars have puzzled over the name Sigerson and uniformly misinterpreted its significance. Holmes's choice of the name has been taken as evidence that Holmes's father was Siger Holmes; hence Sigerson was a tribute to the man who was instrumental in his biological birth. In reality, Holmes had used this name as a tribute to someone who helped in his spiritual rebirth. Why did he not mention Freud at all? Most likely at Freud's request, if not demand, that anything tying Freud to cocaine should be suppressed.

NOTES

All dates in this essay relating to the life of Sherlock Holmes are from the chronological data assembled by William S. Baring-Gould. Further details of this chronology can be found in two publications:
1. Baring-Gould, W. S. (1962): *Sherlock Holmes of Baker Street: A Life of the World's First Consulting Detective.* New York: Bramball House.
2. Baring-Gould, W. S. (1967): *The Annotated Sherlock Holmes.* New York: Potter.
The concept that Sherlock Holmes was a cocaine addict is self-evident from the works of John Watson, M. D., but another physician, David Musto, must be given full credit for first

disseminating this knowledge to the medical world and for first demonstrating the Vienna connection (*JAMA* 204:125–130, 1968). Sigmund Freud's adventures with cocaine are documented in *Cocaine Papers of Sigmund Freud*, edited by Robert Buck (New York: Stonehill, 1974).

Nicholas Monardes's *Joyfull Newes Out of the Newe Founde Worlde* was first published in English in 1577 in the translation by John Frampton. This was last reprinted, to my knowledge, in 1925.

Mary A. B. Brazier's *A History of the Electrical Activity of the Brain* (London: Pitman Medical, 1961) contains a full history of the scramble for authority between Adolf Beck and Ernst Fleischl von Marxow.

Torture in Vienna

It is quite certain that the Jews of every province annually decide by lot which congregation or city is to send Christian blood to the other congregations.

Thomas of Cantimpré (c. 1250)

God will forgive, . . . that's his business.

Heinrich Heine (1797–1856)

Torture in Vienna

Law-enforcement officials have traditionally employed torture for two separate purposes. The first was interrogation, in which torture was used either to obtain self-incriminating evidence (i.e., a confession) or to elicit accusations of putative accomplices. The second purpose was to impose cruel, although not unusual, forms of punishment for criminals, often those who had been convicted on evidence obtained by previous torture.

The Austrian Empire was the last civilized European state to officially sanction torture as a means of gathering evidence. While this policy must have affected the lives of hundreds of thousands, if not millions, of people, the relationship of two physicians to this practice has rarely been told. The two physicians were Solomon Maimon and Ferdinand von Leber, contemporaries who never met and whose lives were as disparate as the ethnic components of the empire in which they lived.

Solomon Maimon was a physician and a philosopher. He was one of the first eastern European Jews to leave the ghetto of his youth to participate in the wider cultural life of western Europe. Today, that insular world of the eastern European ghetto, that was and is no longer, when Jews are an integral part of the intellectual and cultural life throughout the Western world, it is somewhat difficult for us to comprehend how different the situation was a mere 200 years ago. At that time, Jews lived, worked, and studied in a separate world of their own. It was into this world that Maimon was born in 1754, in Niezwicz, in what is now Poland, but was then part of the Austrian Empire. Originally his name was Solomon Ben Joshua, and it was obvious quite early in his life that he was endowed with unusual intellectual ability. At that time in eastern Europe, of course, the only intellectual activity open to Jews was religious learning, and young Solomon soon became well versed in the rabbinic literature. He was married at age 12 to the daughter of a widow from his own town, and by age 14 he was a father. Apparently his mother-in-law was quite oppressive. She continually urged him to go to work, to make a living, so that he could help support his wife, and also, one supposes, his mother-in-law. Solomon Ben Joshua was neither the first nor the last scholar whose intellectual pursuits were hampered by such pragmatic obstacles. For several years he taught religious subjects to various unpromising children, while he himself studied Jewish philosophy. During his studies he was greatly influenced by the writings of Moses Ben Maimon (Maimonides), the great twelfth-century Jewish rabbi, physician, and philosopher, and as a token of his reverence for Maimonides, he assumed the name Maimon.

Maimon soon plunged himself into cabalistic mysticism and attempted to discover its philosophical basis. This irritated the leadership of the Jewish community, who believed that faith, not philosophy, should be the basis of the cabala. Maimon was officially censured, and in his disillusionment he turned to secular studies. In these, as in virtually everything he attempted, he was self-taught.

At last a fortunate accident came to my help. I observed in some stout Hebrew volumes that they contained several alphabets, and that the number of their signatures was indicated not merely by Hebrew letters, but that for this purpose the characters of a second and a third alphabet had also been employed, these being commonly Latin and German. Now I had not the slightest idea of printing. I imagined that books were printed like linen, each page being the impression of a separate form. I presumed, however, that the characters which stood in corresponding places must represent one and the same letter, and as I had already heard something of the order of the alphabet in these languages, I supposed that, for example, a, standing in the same place as aleph, must likewise be an aleph in sound. In this way I gradually learnt the Latin and German characters.

By a kind of deciphering I began to combine various German letters into words; but as the characters corresponding to the Hebrew letters might be something quite different from the Hebrew, I was always in doubt whether the whole of my labor in this operation might not be in vain, till fortunately some leaves of an old German book fell into my hand. I began to read. How great were my joy and surprise when I saw from the connection, that the words completely corresponded with what I had learned. In my Jewish language, to be sure, many of the words were unintelligible; but from the context I was still able, even omitting such words, to comprehend the whole pretty well.

This mode of learning by deciphering still constitutes my peculiar method of comprehending and judging the thoughts of others. I maintain that no one can say he understands a book as long as he finds himself compelled to deliver the author's thoughts in the order and connection determined by the author, and with the expressions which he has used. This is a mere work of note, and no man can flatter himself with having comprehended an author till he is roused by his thoughts, which he apprehends at first but dimly, to reflect on the subject himself, and to work it out for himself, though it may be under the impulse of another. This distinction between different kinds of understanding must be evident to any man of discernment. For the same reason also I can understand a book only when the thoughts which it contains harmonize after the intervening gaps are filled out.

Starting in this manner, he went on to study physics and finally medicine, and he even became, in his own words, "a physician." Maimon described his rigorous medical education as follows:

From my generous friend, the chief rabbi, I subsequently received two medical works, Kulm's Anatomical Tables and Voit's Gaziopilatium. The latter is a large medical dictionary, containing, in brief form, not only explanations in all departments of medicine, but also their manifold applications. In connection with every disease explanations of its cause, symptoms, and the method of its cure are given, along with the ordinary prescriptions. This was a real treasure. I studied the book thoroughly, and believed myself to be master of the science of medicine and a complete physician.

But I was not going to content myself with mere theory in this matter; I resolved to make regular application of it. I visited patients, determined all diseases according to their circumstances and symptoms, explained their causes, and also gave prescriptions for their cure. But in this practice things turned out very comically. If a patient told me some of the symptoms of his disease, I deduced the nature of the disease itself, and inferred the presence of other symptoms. If the patient said that he could feel none of these, I stubbornly insisted on their being present all the same. Our conversation sometimes came to this:

I. "You have a headache also."

Patient. "No."

I. "But you must have a headache."

As many symptoms are common in several diseases, I frequently took quid pro quo. Prescriptions I could never keep in my head, so that when I was to prescribe anything, I was obliged to go home first and turn up my Gaziopilatium. At length I even began to make up drugs myself according to Voit's prescriptions. How this succeeded may be imagined. It had at least this good result, that I saw something more surely required for a practical physician than I understood at the time.

As his studies progressed, his thirst for knowledge grew, and he finally left for Germany. His various adventures and misadventures in western Europe are too complex to detail here. He never formally studied medicine, never supported himself by practicing medicine, and never really made a living in any occupation. However, he did become a noted philosopher. His work was admired by Kant, Goethe, Schiller, and others, and his writings were a major influence in nineteenth-century German philosophy and intellectual life. His autobiography, from which the preceding quotations are taken, was published in 1793. This work remains a major document for this period in regard to spiritual and intellectual ferment. Among his early recollections was the following story:

My grandfather, Heimann Joseph, held the lease of certain villages in the estates of Prince Radzivil, in the neighborhood of the town of Mir. The Papa, that is the Russian cleric of Mir, was a stupid and ignorant clod, barely able to read and write. Most of his time he spent at the tavern, drinking with his boorish parishioners, and he always had his liquor charged to his account, with never a thought of paying his score. Grandfather (who owned the tavern) at last wearied of this, and determined to extend no further credit. As was expected, the man took umbrage, and meditated vengeance.

Eventually he hit upon a device, frightful indeed in the eyes of humanity, but one of which Catholic Christians in the Poland of the period were wont to make frequent use. His scheme was to charge my grandfather with the murder of a Christian, and so compass his death by judicial hanging. The circumstances were as follows. A beaver trapper who hunted the region for the game which was to be taken on the Niemen sometimes sold his catch to my grandfather; this had to be done secretly for beavers are a royal preserve, and all that are taken must be delivered to the court. Once the trapper came about midnight, knocked, and had grandfather summoned. He displayed a bag, quite heavy to lift, and said with mysterious air: "I have brought you a stout fellow here." Grandfather wished to strike a light, examine the beaver, and dicker for it with the trapper. But the trapper said there was no need: grandfather could take the beaver, and they would be sure to agree upon terms afterwards. Grandfather suspected no evil, and so took the sack just as it was, laid it aside, and again betook himself to rest. But he had scarcely fallen asleep when he was again aroused by loud knocking.

It was the priest, with some boors from the village, who at once began to make a thorough search. They found the sack, and grandfather was terrified, though he could suspect no worse than that he had been informed against on account of his clandestine traffic in beavers and would be in a position to protest innocence. But how great was his horrow when the sack was opened and instead of a beaver a human corpse came to view!

Straightaway grandfather's hands were bound behind his back, his feet were put into stocks, he was cast into a cart, brought to the town of Mir, and there delivered to the criminal court. He was made fast in fetters and thrust into a dungeon. At the trial my grandfather insisted upon his innocence, related the events exactly as they transpired, and, reasonably enough, demanded that the trapper too should be examined. But the trapper was nowhere to be found; he was already over the hills and far away. A search was instituted, but the bloodthirsty judge found the delay tedious, and thrice running ordered grandfather subjected to torture. Grandfather persisted in his claim that he was innocent of murder.

At last the trapper was discovered. He was examined, and as he denied the whole affair straightway, he was subjected to trial by torture, whereupon his story tumbled forth. He declared he had found the dead body in the water some time previously, and had wished to fetch it to the parsonage for burial. But the priest had said to him: "There is time enough for burial. You know that the Jews are stubborn people, and hence damned to all eternity. They have crucified our Lord Jesus Christ, and to this day they seek Christian blood, if they can manage to obtain any, for use at their Passover festival, which they have instituted as a mark of their triumph. They use the blood for their Passover loaves. You will be performing a meritorious deed if you can smuggle this dead body into the house of that accursed Jew of a leaseholder. You will of course have to clear out, but then in your trade you can drive anywhere." Upon this confession the fellow was whipped and my grandfather set free; but the priest continued as priest.

An official governmental accusation that a Jew had killed a Christian in order to use his blood for ritual purposes in eastern Europe in the middle of the eighteenth century may seem surprising. It should not. After all, accusations of this nature had been a part of European culture for centuries. Such a blood libel or blood accusation was based on the mistaken belief that the Jewish religion required periodic ritualistic consumption of the blood of Christians. The most frequent accusation was that Jews murdered children in order to obtain blood that was needed to make unleavened bread (matzo) for Passover. This type of calumny against Jews was born in the Middle Ages, at about the time of the First Crusade. The Jews were not the first religious minority to be unjustly accused of this crime by members of the majority, who neither understood the Jewish religion nor cared enough to try to understand it. A thousand years earlier, Christians had been accused of the same crime by the Romans. But by the Middle Ages the Christians were the accusers, and their memory did not go back to Roman times. It is believed that a Jew named Young William, of Norwich, England, who died in 1144, was the first victim to be executed as a direct result of a blood accusation. Once started, such accusations continued to recur across the centuries.

Visitors to the cathedral in Lincoln, England, can see the tomb of "Little St. Hugh" an alleged victim of a ritual murder. Eight-year-old Hugh of Lincoln disappeared on July 31, 1255, and his body was discovered one month later in a well at the house of a Jew named Joscefin or Jopin. On the promise of having his life spared, Jopin was induced by a priest, John of Lexington, to admit that the innocent Christian boy had been crucified by a group of prominent Jews from many parts of England who were then gathered in Lincoln for a wedding. The remains of the boy were then buried in the cathedral with great ceremony. One month later, King Henry III visited Lincoln, revoked Jopin's pardon, and had Jopin dragged around the city tied to a wild horse and then hung. The other 92 Jews in Lincoln were taken to London, where 18 of them were pressed to death while refusing to enter a plea. The others remained in prison until Richard, earl of Cornwall, who according to feudal law possessed all Jews in England, arranged for their release. The crown confiscated the property of all those executed and exacted a ransom for the others. The church thus gained a martyr, whose shrine can still be seen. Even Chaucer was impressed by the event and referred to it at the beginning of *The Prioress' Tale*.

Blood accusations were never official church policy. The hierarchy of the Roman Catholic church always understood that such charges had no basis in fact. This, of course, did little good. Denunciation of the practice by four different popes (Innocent IV in 1247, Gregory X in 1272, Martin V in 1422, and Paul III in 1457) did not prevent recurrences of such trumped-up charges. There were numerous instances during the nineteenth century in such diverse locales as Russia, Hungary, and Syria. The latter involved Jews of Damascus who were charged with drinking the blood of an elderly Syrian Christian monk. Heinrich Heine, the great German-Jewish poet, on hearing the details of this case, is said to have remarked, "Chacun a son gout." Heine's disdain for such charges was typical of the reaction of educated people in his day, Jews and non-Jews alike. No one with any degree of sophistication believed that such ridiculous charges deserved a serious answer. The disdain of intellectuals had even less influence than the denunciation of popes. Blood libels continued, both as acts of irrational bigotry by half-crazed zealots and as official government policy in some areas. The accusation made against Maimon's grandfather combined both of these elements. But it was not the act of a reactionary government led by a paranoid anti-Semite; it was an official charge of the Austrian Empire and the established church through its local representative. This was not the last time a European government made such an accusation. The most famous of all blood accusations occurred in Kiev, Russia, in September 1913, when the Imperial Russian government brought charges against Mendel Beiliss that he had murdered a Christian boy in order to use his blood for ritual purposes as demanded by the Jewish religion. If this could happen in Russia in 1913, it is easy to imagine it occurring in the backwaters of the Austrian Empire over 200 years earlier.

History thus makes it clear that we should not be at all taken aback by the nature of the charge made against Maimon's grandfather. The use of torture is another question. The fact that the Austrian judiciary still employed torture in criminal proceeds, on the other hand is truly a subject for wonderment. After all, blood libels were known as late as the twentieth century, but the use of torture is popularly believed to have ended in Europe with the Middle Ages. The practice of using torture to extract evidence from those accused of crimes was widespread during the Middle Ages; in fact, it was part of the legal code in virtually every European country. In most countries it was part of the heritage left behind by the Roman conquerors. In Italy, France, and Germany, the use of torture during questioning of accused criminals can be traced directly to Roman times. In various times and places the type and severity of the torture varied, but the concept remained un-challenged.

In England, the rack was introduced as a device for torture, as well as for punishment, in the reign of Henry VI. Other forms of torture were employed in England at various times, including the "scavenger's daughter," an appliance that drew the head and feet together, after which the prisoner was left on the floor either to confess or eventually to die. Prisoners who refused to plead had their bodies pressed with iron weights until they either entered a plea or died. The 18 Jews accused of crucifying Hugh of Lincoln died in this way. This remained common legal practice until the reign of George III. In Scotland, the iron boot was used for torture. The prisoner's foot was crowded into this receptacle, and iron wedges were driven in at the sides until the foot was crushed. This method was used chiefly to settle differences in ecclesiastical opinion and to convince the victim of religious truths.

To a large extent the use of torture had died out in England before the founding of the English colonies in the New World. The best-known and most widely practiced form of torture in New England was the dunking stool. This was used exclusively for the purpose of extracting information from those accused of crimes. However, there are records in early Massachusetts archives of a Giles Corey who underwent torture during the witch trials in Salem. He was slowly pressed to death after he had refused to plead.

The use of torture was part of the legacy of Rome, but Christian Europe built on this legacy. The uncertainties and stresses of life in the Middle Ages were factors contributing to the spread of the practice of trial by torture. During this period, wave after wave of plague, such as the Black Death in England, France, Germany, and eastern Europe and the sweating sickness in middle and southern Europe, depopulated towns and cities and even entire countries. Whereas some attributed such plagues to supernatural causes, others believed that human hands had brought on these disasters. Many people, both Jewish and Christian, were accused of poisoning water wells and were subjected to torture, even tortured to death if they failed to name their imaginary accomplices. In the extremity of their suffering many such prisoners were driven to make false accusations and were for a time relieved of their torture, but in nearly all instances they were finally burned. The Jewish population in these countries suffered especially, many of them being burned to death, each one of them first having been subjected to torture in order to obtain the names of supposed accomplices. Thus the Jews of eastern Europe certainly were not strangers to the danger of being tortured to confess to crimes of which they could not possibly be guilty.

Legal torture was practiced in France during the reigns of the various kings Louis, primarily the process of drawing and quartering, although this was used more for punishment than to obtain information. In this procedure, horses pulled ropes attached to the prisoner's four limbs. The object, of course, was to pull the limbs from the body. If the horses failed in this, the torture chief would use a long knife to sever the limbs from the body. This method of inflicting punishment was a part of the legal code of France until the time of Napoleon.

Although such cruel punishments for those convicted of crimes persisted until the nineteenth century, the use of torture as an investigative tool had generally disappeared much earlier. This was not the case in the Austrian Empire of Solomon Maimon's time. There, under Empress Maria Theresa, the torturing of suspects continued unabated.

Illiteracy was the common condition even long after the Middle Ages, and many of those involved in the process of torture either as victim or executioner were unable to read. To overcome this handicap, drawings were prepared to demonstrate how torture should be conducted. A number of these drawings still survive from the reign of Maria Theresa of Austria, showing the various methods of manipulating torture implements.

The artists employed by Maria Theresa's government were expert in making their pictures explicitly explain everything that was expected to the ignorant mind of the chief torturer. One such drawing shows the thumbscrew, in which the thumbs of the victim were placed between crossbars of iron with sharp points. It is obvious from the drawing that the lever can be turned so as to bring the iron bars closer together and drive the sharp points into the thumbs of the victim. This minor torture was used only to suggest what would follow if the prisoner failed to confess at once.

Another sketch from the *Constitutio Criminalis Theresiana* depicts the method of using the rack and the burning candle. One can easily understand from this drawing how the contrivance could be most effectively employed. First the prisoner was placed on his back on a ladderlike appliance. His arms were bound to a rung of the ladder. His legs were then connected by ropes to a cylinder, which was turned by an assistant until gradually the prisoner's shoulders and knees were dislocated. During this process the operator was to apply a lighted candle to the armpits. This famous document depicts other tortures that were even more horrible, the descriptions of which I shall spare the reader. These drawings were used both to enlighten the torturer and to frighten the accused.

A major question, of course, is how frequently these devices were actually used. In Austria at the time of Maria Theresa, no one accused of a crime was allowed to testify in his own behalf, nor could others testify for him until they had been subjected to torture.

It was through the influence of two contemporaries of Maimon (one an Austrian physician, the other a converted Jew) that Austria, the last European nation to officially sanction torture, was finally freed from this vestige of the Middle Ages. The first of these men was Ferdinand von Leber; the second was Joseph von Sonnenfels. Leber was born in Vienna in 1727, the son of a wigmaker and a wet-nurse. As a Catholic, Leber was able to take full advantage of the educational and career opportunities the Austrian Empire offered. In contrast to Maimon, Leber was a fully trained physician, having received his degree from the University of Vienna in 1751. Following his graduation, he became associated with the hospital at Breitenfurt and soon became recognized as a skillful surgeon. When his former professor died in 1761, Leber was given the position of Professor of Anatomy and

Theoretical Surgery at the University of Vienna. During his time at the university he did much to upgrade the curriculum and also was active in adding to the pathology museum. In 1786 he gave up the teaching of anatomy so that he could concentrate on surgery, especially on his interest in improving the design of surgical instruments. In 1776 he had been named private surgeon to Empress Maria Theresa. In 1805, after 41 years of public service, he was given a gold medal by Emporer Francis I for his outstanding contributions. He died in 1808 of a stroke.

For 19 years, from 1757 until 1776, Leber held the position of *Folterarzt*, or torture physician. In this position, one of Leber's duties was to examine prisoners to determine whether or nor they were amenable to torture, that is, whether they would be more likely to survive torture or to die. After all, if torture is the appropriate way to examine the accused, an unintended death during the procedure would unbalance the scales of justice. In this capacity he learned, as many others must also have discovered before him, that innocent defendants often confess to the most impossible acts in order to avoid further pain. When he became convinced of the truth of this observation, he decided, despite the obvious risks, to try to get such legal torture abolished in Austria and all the Hapsburg lands, including Hungary, Galicia, and Poland.

During Leber's tenure as torture physician, two particularly perplexing cases were heard in the Vienna court. These involved two suspects named Eleanor Kermin and Franz Sachs. No satisfactory confession of guilt had been obtained from either of the accused by the ordinary methods of torture. In such a situation, the law provided for a more severe form of interrogation called intercalary torture. This form of torture was expressly prescribed by the *Constitutio Criminalis Theresiana*:

> It is first ordained that ordinarily the torture should be completed, one step after the other, in one day; secondly, as it is often the case that those who have been previously tortured for other misdeeds, or are of an especially strong state of body, or are evil doers of long practice, are insensitive to the torture practised in this way and the truth cannot be elicited from them, for such wicked people, at the decision of the upper court, as an exceptional case, the torture may be extended over two or three days.

In practice, this meant that torture almost to the point of death would be applied on three successive days. Dr. Leber, who was aghast at normal torture procedures, did not believe that anyone should be subjected to this extreme form of interrogation. Sachs was the first of the suspects to undergo intercalary torture, and the first day of interrogation/torture went by without anything out of the ordinary having been noted. Leber, as his position demanded, examined Sachs. Following his examination, Leber, in conjunction with another local surgeon named Wober, declared that Sachs was physically capable of being tortured, medically speaking, but that despite this, Sachs should not be tortured again until he had completely recovered from the initial day of interrogation. The two physicians, with Leber taking the lead, went even further than this and declared that the three days of torture should never be given on consecutive days, that all suspects should be allowed to mend fully before undergoing torture again. The die was cast. Leber had challenged the legal establishment and governmental authorities. The establishment decided to go over Leber's head to a higher medical authority and turned to the entire medical faculty of the University of Vienna. The medical faculty, of which Leber was a respected and influential member, supported Leber's views. They declared that intercalary torture should not be used in this case or any other case until the suspect was fully healed.

The medical faculty declared "that while a prisoner is only taken to be tortured after he has been found healthy and fit by the surgeon, on the other hand, a prisoner, who has had the thumbscrews and the first band of the press applied on the previous day, develops inflammatory swelling, so that he becomes unfit for a further intercalated torture. Furthermore, gangrene can easily follow in the already inflamed parts." The faculty therefore unanimously decided that torture with thumbscrew, press, and rack should be practiced without danger to life and only on a prisoner with a proper constitution, never three days in succession or with only a three-day interval. Finally, in the specific case of Franz Sachs, the faculty applied its own rules and stated that intercalary torture should not be completed.

This relatively mild statement, which called for only a limited modification of the overall practice of torture, caused a furor. The entire question of torture itself as a means of examining suspects began to be challenged. Finally the question was brought up in front of the Viennese version of the bar, and its decision was in favor of retaining the existing practices. The cases of Sachs and Kermin were still undecided, and Leber finally sought a personal audience with the empress herself. In an apparently emotional appeal Leber pleaded with Maria Theresa to declare a verdict without requiring repeated and severe torture. Maria Theresa granted his request, and the prisoners were acquitted. Soon the empress, with further urging from Leber, Sonnenfels, and other humanists, made this decree: "The findings of the medical faculty move me to abolish the intercalated torture absolutely." The Austrian legal profession, instead of welcoming this advancement from the practices of the Middle Ages, were angry with Leber for interfering with what they considered their special prerogative. It was demanded that Leber be expelled from the capital. Threats were also made against his life, but it appears that there was no actual attempt to murder him, and he continued in his role as court physician, although of course he no longer had to examine potential candidates for intercalary torture.

The cases of Eleanor Kermin and Franz Sachs were quite famous in their time, having implications as important as those of the Dreyfus case in France and the Leopold and Loeb case in the United States. The publicity and resulting change in public opinion these cases provoked led to the final abolishment of all forms of torture as means of obtaining evidence within the Austrian Empire.

Joseph Edler von Sonnenfels played a major role in influencing government officials and the public to support a total ban on all torture. Sonnenfels was the son of Perlin Lipmann Sonnenfels, a noted Austrian scholar, who in turn was the son of the chief rabbi of Brandenburg. Early in his adult life, Lipmann had left Brandenburg and obtained employment in the princely house of Dietrickstein at Nicholsburg, where his son Joseph was born in 1732. Sometime between 1735 and

1741 he and his children converted to Catholicism and moved to Vienna. There Lipmann became a teacher of Semitic languages at the University of Vienna and an official Hebrew translator for the courts. He was knighted in 1746 and given the name Sonnenfels. His son Joseph studied philosophy at the University of Vienna and then served several years in the army. He received his law degree in 1754 and began a successful law practice in Vienna. In 1763 he became professor of political sciences at the university. His widely read essay on torture was published in 1776, and the next year all forms of torture were finally banned throughout the Austrian Empire.

Three years later Joseph von Sonnenfels was given the rank of court councillor to the Austrian chancellery, and in 1810 he became president of the Imperial Academy of Sciences, a position he held until his death in 1817. Throughout his life he was active as a novelist and critic. His *Letters on the Viennese Stage* helped reform the theater in Vienna, which had been dominated by burlesque clowns and buffoonish caricatures of Jews and other minority groups. He worked hard to promote an atmosphere of toleration for all non-Catholics in Austria, and at the same time he helped to infuse the press with a spirit of boldness and freedom. He helped create the Vienna that Goethe called "the capital of our fatherland, when the dawn is breaking for its most beautiful day." Sonnenfels is perhaps best remembered today because a fellow resident of his beloved Vienna, Ludwig van Beethoven, dedicated to Sonnenfels the Pastoral Sonata in D Major.

Maimon, who had already left Austria, was unaware of the events that were occurring there. He still had no job. Because his mind fed on a combination of metaphysical problems and alcohol, he was not suited for any practical occupation. In 1790 he was finally given asylum by Count Kalkreuth on his estate at Niedersiegerdorf, Germany, where Maimon died in 1800. Maimon concluded his story about his grandfather as follows:

> For an everlasting memorial of grandfather's deliverance from death, my father composed in Hebrew a sort of epic poem interspersed with songs, in which the narrative of the whole event was related and God's goodness celebrated. The rule was established that the day of deliverance should be celebrated in the family annually, and that at this celebration the poem should be recited, just as the Book of Esther is read at the Purim festival.

If anyone still celebrates this festival, let us hope that they have added a song in honor of Dr. Leber, whose achievements are otherwise little remembered.

NOTES

The autobiography of Solomon Maimon was first published in German in 1793. The English translation quoted here, by J. Clark Murray, professor of mental and moral philosophy at McGill University, was published in London in 1888. A version edited by Moses Hadas is still available (*Solomon Maimon*, edited by Moses Hadas. New York: Schocken Books). The best source for biographical material on Maimon and Sonnenfels and historical data on blood libels remains the *Jewish Encyclopaedia*, edited by Isidore Singer and published by Funk & Wagnalls. The story of the role of Ferdinand von Leber in the abolishment of torture in Austria can be found in Dr. Donald T. Atkinson's *Magic, Myth, and Medicine* and in Max Neuberger's *Essays in the History of Medicine* (New York: Medical Life Press, 1930).

The twentieth-century Russian blood libel is recorded in Maurice Samuels's *The Blood Accusation*. This was also used by Bernard Malamud as the basis of his novel *The Fixer*.

The Names Behind the Eponyms

How is it that one fine morning Duchenne discovered a disease that probably existed in the time of Hippocrates?

J. M. Charcot

You can observe a lot just by watching.

Edward (Yogi) Berra

The Names Behind the Eponyms

Joseph François Felix Babinski (1857–1932)

Eighty years ago Joseph Babinski (Fig. 1) described the reflex of dorsiflexion of the great toe on stimulation of the sole of the foot. This brief but historic report consisted of only 28 lines and was given at a meeting of the Société de Biologie de Paris, February 22, 1896. Entitled "On the cutaneous plantar reflex in certain organic affections of the central nervous system," Babinski's report was as follows:

> In a certain number of cases of hemiplegia or crural monoplegia associated with an organic affection of the central nervous system, I have observed a perturbation in the cutaneous plantar reflex of which the following is a brief description: On the healthy side, pricking the plantar surface of the foot provokes, as is usual in

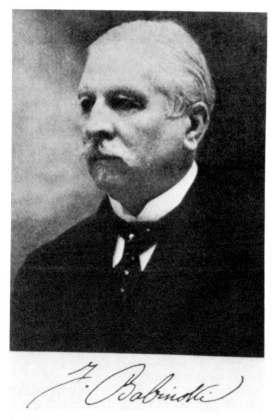

FIG. 1. Photograph of Joseph Babinski, late in life (From Webb Haymaker, *The Founders of Neurology*, 1953. Courtesy of Charles C Thomas, Springfield, Ill.)

the normal state, flexion of the thigh on the pelvis, of the leg and of the toes on the metatarsus. On the paralyzed side a similar excitation gives rise also to flexion of the thigh on the pelvis, of the leg on the thigh, and of the foot on the leg; but the toes instead of flexing, execute a movement of extension on the metatarsus. I have observed this disturbance in cases of recent hemiplegia of only a few days duration, as well as in cases of spastic hemiplegia that had existed for several months; I have demonstrated it in patients who were incapable of voluntary movement of the toes and also in subjects who could still execute voluntary movement of the toes; but I must add that this disturbance is not constant. I have also observed in a number of cases of crural paraplegia due to an organic lesion of the cord a movement of extension of the toes following pricking the sole of the foot.

The fact that stimulation of the sole of the foot could elicit dorsiflexion of the great toe had been described by E. Remak 3 years earlier, but Babinski was the first to realize the significance of this phenomenon. It is appropriate that this reflex carries Babinski's name rather than Remak's name, because it was not the discovery of the phenomenon but the discovery of its meaning that was significant. Newton was not the first to discover that apples fall down from apple trees.

No other single presentation has ever had as great an influence on the field of neurology as this report. In its simplicity, clinical importance, and physiological implications, this reflex probably has no equal. However, the Babinski reflex did not immediately receive international recognition. Babinski himself contributed two more reports that further elucidated the phenomenon. The first, "On the phenomenon of toes and its semeiotic value," appeared in *La Semaine Medicale* in 1898. After a relatively long discussion of his personal experience with the new reflex in a variety of neurologic conditions, Babinski stated:

My observations have demonstrated that the toe phenomenon can be caused by a disturbance of the pyramidal system, whatever its duration, intensity, and extent. I have observed it in very old as well as in rather recent cases of hemiplegia, in cases where the nerve fibers of the pyramidal tract had been destroyed and in others (due to sclerotic plagues, for instance) where the alteration was only slight or the axis cylinders of this tract were preserved. In some subjects the lesions of the tract were very extensive and in others the lesions were limited. It is worthwhile to note that this sign, although it indicates the presence of a pyramidal system disturbance, does not denote its severity. . . . At times it can even be the only sign indicating such a disturbance.

Babinski's next contribution was again a short note, "On the abduction of the toes," which appeared in *Revue Neurologique* in 1903. This report contained the first description of abduction of the toes on stimulation of the sole of the foot:

More recently observed facts have led me to think that such a lesion could also effect an associated abduction of the toes. To witness this phenomenon, the following conditions must be observed: the subject lies on his back, then having crossed his arms across his chest, performs alternate movements of flexion and extension of the trunk over the pelvis, as in the research of the "combined movement of flexion of the trunk and of the thigh." While he performs these acts, the toes will spread apart.
The associated abduction of the toes seems to have a clinical significance of the same order as does the reflex abduction, but it must be noted that if these two

types of movements sometimes coexist, one may also exist in the absence of the other.

Associated abduction of the toes is a rather rare phenomenon that seems to me to be more common to infantile hemiplegia than in that of the adult, more frequent in hemiparesis than in hemiplegia.

An article in *Revue Neurologique* in 1900, by two French neurologists whose names are best not recorded, stated that the diagnostic value of the Babinski reflex was quite minimal, and even the great Oppenheim initially maintained that a toe reflex would never gain any great importance in neurologic diagnosis. Oppenheim, of course, reversed his position and with great fanfare introduced his own toe reflex a few years later (1902). Despite detractors and all those who described minor variations to which they or others attached their names, Babinski's contribution was pivotal and soon brought him world renown.

Much like proud parents, countries bask in reflected glory because of the accomplishments of their famous offspring. Because national origin frequently is a more complex issue than even biological parentage, some individuals of sufficient prestige are claimed by more than one fatherland or motherland. Such is the case with Joseph Babinski, whose memory is cherished by three claimants: France, Poland, and Argentina. In fact, it has even been claimed that he was born in each of these three locations. France and Poland are obvious, but how did Argentina get involved? Babinski's parents left Poland after the political upheaval in 1848. Like many other political refugees of that era, they were not welcomed anywhere in Europe. They fled to the New World, arriving in Argentina. Like many other political activists of their time, the Babinski family returned to Europe when the political climate shifted. Thus it was that Babinski, of Polish descent, was born in Paris after having been conceived in Argentina. The claim that he was both conceived and born in Argentina cannot be substantiated.

Babinski's father was an engineer. His mother was an educated woman who was dedicated to the education of Joseph and his older brother Henri. The family lived on the Left Bank, near the ancient abbey of St-Germain-des-Pres. Henri enrolled in L'Ecole des Mines, and Joseph entered the medical school of the University of Paris.

Joseph graduated in 1884, and his thesis, "Etude anatomique et clinique sur la sclerose en plagues," was a pioneer contribution to the study of multiple sclerosis and was one of the first attempts to correlate the clinical and pathological findings in this disorder. That same year, Charcot, with whom Babinski had not yet worked, had an unexpected vacancy in the post of chief of clinic because of the sudden death of one of his interns. The position of Chef de Clinique a la Faculté de Medecine at that time was the first significant step up the academic ladder. On completion of an internship of 1 to 4 years, a prospective academician was eligible for appointment as a chief of clinic under a faculty professor. The appointment was made by the professor and was not determined by any competitive examination. The two leading candidates were Babinski, who had interned in neurology with Vulpian, and a contemporary of Babinski named Richardiere. At the time the unexpected vacancy occurred, these two were competing in an international medical competition. It was suggested to Charcot that he give the appointment to the loser, and Charcot agreed. Thus Richardiere won the competition, and as far as I know was never heard from again. Babinski lost and became chief of clinic at the Salpetriere under Charcot (Fig. 2).

The next advance for Babinski was the position Medecine des Hôpitaux de Paris (physician of the hospitals of Paris). This post was granted only after a competitive examination. To be eligible to take this examination, a candidate had to have been chief of clinic for at least 2 years. Babinski became Medecine des Hôpitaux de Paris in 1890 and was appointed to the staff of Hôpital de la Pitíe, with which he remained associated for the rest of his career.

The penultimate academic appointment was Professor Agrege a la Faculté de Medecine (professor of the aggregation in the faculty of medicine). This prestigious title is based on a very difficult competitive examination that only few pass. Charcot himself was not successful the first time he took the examination. Babinski was a candidate in 1892, and another protégé of Charcot, Bouchard, was presiding over the examination. Bouchard had been an intern under Charcot, as well as a collaborator with Charcot. But Bouchard's main interests by 1892 were his own department and his own protégés. Bouchard managed to have Babinski eliminated in favor of his own candidate. As a result, Babinski, one of the greatest clinical teachers of his day, never had a formal teaching position in the faculty of medicine of Paris.

Babinski's scientific writings ranged widely, from his first paper on typhoid fever, written in 1882, to his last contribution on hysteria, which appeared in 1930. All of his work after 1890 was confined to clinical neurology.

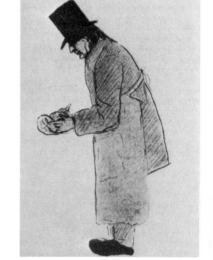

FIG. 2.   Sketch of J. M. Charcot examining a brain in the amphitheater of Salpetriere, by Brissaud.

While memorialized by his famous sign, Babinski made many other significant contributions to neurology. His analysis of cerebellar symptomatology is the basis of much of our understanding of this topic and laid the foundation for the concept of asynergy as the underlying symptom of cerebellar dysfunction. He first described the loss of the pupillary response to light in cerebral syphilis. He described a patient with dystrophia adiposogenitalis the year before Fröhlich did. He and Nageotte were largely responsible for recognizing the physiological basis of locomotor ataxia, and they gave the first correct explanation of the loss of deep tendon reflexes in this disorder.

Babinski believed that his major contribution was not his description of the toe reflex but his role in the development of neurosurgery in France. In 1922 he localized the first spinal cord tumor to be operated on successfully in France. He enthusiastically urged surgical exploration of brain tumors, and he was instrumental in inducing two of his students, de Martel and Clovis Vincent, to become neurosurgeons and develop neurosurgery in France.

Hysteria had been a major interest of Charcot, and it was only natural that this interest was shared by his students, including Sigmund Freud and Joseph Babinski. Babinski devoted a great deal of time and energy to the study of hysteria and related conditions. Robert Wartenberg, in an article in the *Journal of the American Medical Association* (135:763–767, 1947) entitled "The Babinski Reflex after Fifty Years," related that he had asked Babinski how he had actually discovered the reflex. Babinski told Wartenberg that like other neurologists he had been concerned primarily with the differential diagnosis of organic and hysterical hemiplegia and had wanted to find some reflex or behavior that would be helpful. The Babinski reflex was the result of this investigation. It is interesting that Babinski made the same use of abduction of the toes (*Revue Neurologique* 11:728–729, 1903):

> Recently, in a case of crural paraplegia due to trauma, which motivated a medico-legal evaluation, the physicians charged with the examination were of the opinion that they were dealing with hysteria or malingering because the classical objective signs of organic disease of the nervous system were absent. Having observed in this patient a very distinct abduction of the toes, I gave a contrary opinion. About three weeks after my first consultation, a second examination permitted me to demonstrate an extension of the toes which had not been found previously and which confirmed my view.

Babinski's concept of hysteria was rejected in his time and is now virtually forgotten. He employed the term *pithiatisme*, which was constructed from the Greek words for persuasion and curable. He believed that hysteria was produced by suggestion and could be abolished by suggestion and was not primarily triggered by emotional conflict. During World War I he continued his work on war neuroses, and both his critics and enthusiasts agreed that he was more successful in treating such patients than any other practitioner in France.

Charles Gilbert Chaddock (1861–1936) is perhaps the best remembered of Babinski's protégés. Chaddock was an assistant to Babinski at La Pitíe from 1897 to 1899. He then returned to the United States and became professor of nervous and mental diseases at Marion-Sims College, which later became St. Louis University. From 1902 to 1921 Chaddock frequently returned to Paris to work with Babinski, who was both his mentor and his close friend. Chaddock translated several of Babinski's papers for English publication. These appeared in 1914 in the *Interstate Medical Journal* under the title "Selected Works of Joseph Babinski." Chaddock had described his variation of the Babinski reflex in the same journal 3 years earlier. Few neurologists who apply a stimulus to the skin beneath the external malleolus and then attach Chaddock's name to what they have done realize the direct descent of this "new" diagnostic sign.

Never marrying, Joseph Babinski shared living quarters throughout his life with his brother Henri. Henri was a successful mining engineer, a world traveler, a noted gourmet, and author of a famous cookbook, *Gastronomie Pratique*. This guide to gourmet cuisine, which traces the development of gastronomy from antiquity through the early twentieth century, was published under the pseudonym Ali-Bab. Pearce Bailey has suggested that this may stand for other (Ali) Babinski (Bab). In this day of fast foods, Henri's noted observation on American eating habits remains cogent:

> One cannot reproach the inhabitants of the United [States] for living in order to eat; most of them hardly take enough time to even swallow food rapidly; under these conditions it is difficult for a culinary art to develop. . . . The newly arrived are immediately absorbed into the struggle for life, those who have already arrived are preoccupied unceasingly with a defense of their positions, and it is rare to find philosophers who can spare time to enjoy food. . . . I saw on the Stock Exchange in Wall Street millionaires standing up to eat a lunch of corned beef and pickles or a sandwich. I pitied them.

Joseph Babinski was one of the founding members of the Societé de Neurologie de Paris. For many years he was an editor of *Revue Neurologique*. He was active in the development of neurology in Poland, and he presided over the first congress of Polish neurologists, psychiatrists, and psychologists in Warsaw in 1909. In 1914 he was elected to the French Academy of Medicine, and in 1924 he was elected an honorary member of the American Neurological Association.

To the noted American neurophysiologist and medical historian Joseph Fulton, Babinski was one of the few physicians who restricted themselves to clinical medicine and still made significant contributions to both clinical neurology and basic neurophysiology. Babinski's life and work demonstrate that research need not be confined to the laboratory.

The last few years of Babinski's life were complicated by severe Parkinson disease. He died in his beloved Paris in 1932, and his passing was noted in many more than just three countries. The feelings of the world community of neurologists toward this great clinician and teacher were perhaps best expressed in 1913 at the Second International Medical Congress in London, where he received a much-deserved standing ovation. If eponyms are perpetuated as a way of paying homage to the memory of illustrious predecessors who have contributed to the development of clinical neurology, then there is no justification for ever replacing Babinski's name with the anatomic term *plantar*. After all, that already denotes a variety of warts.

Hermann Oppenheim (1858–1919)

Two separate and different distinctions belong to Oppenheim (Fig. 3). He was the leader of German neurology during the latter part of the nineteenth century and the early part of the twentieth century. In fact, his textbook *Lehrbuch der Nervenkrankheiten* is considered to have been a significant landmark in the development of neurology. He was also the first German-born neurologist to feel the effects of the official government anti-Semitism in his native land. Born in Warburg, Westphalia, he studied medicine at three leading German universities: Göttingen, Berlin, and Bonn. After graduation, he became an assistant first at a psychiatric clinic in Berlin and then at the neurologic and psychiatric clinic at the Charité, Berlin's largest hospital and part of the University of Berlin. There he studied with Carl Westphal (1833–1890), who is perhaps best remembered today for a description of the nucleus he shares eponymously with Edinger, but who should be honored by clinicians for his original description of the knee jerk in 1875. Westphal, as professor of psychiatry, made numerous fundamental contributions to neurology,

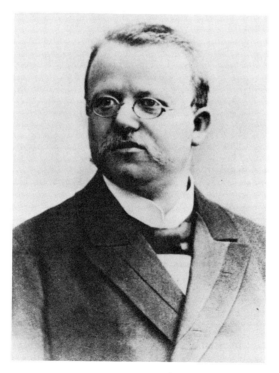

FIG. 3. Photograph of Hermann Oppenheim. (From Lawrence C. McHenry, *Garrison's History of Neurology*, 1969. Courtesy of Charles C Thomas, Springfield, Ill.)

and his neurology clinic was perhaps the leading one in Germany, challenged only by Erb's clinic in Leipzig. Beginning as an assistant, Oppenheim soon became Westphal's associate and he actually took charge during Westphal's long terminal illness. Following Westphal's death, Oppenheim was not given Westphal's position of professor at the Charité; instead, he was forced to leave that august institution and open his own private clinic. This was a direct result of government anti-Semitism. On Westphal's death, the medical faculty of the University of Berlin had unanimously nominated Oppenheim to succeed Westphal as Professor Extraordinarius, a nomination that the Prussian secretary of education adamantly refused to confirm.

Despite such difficulties, Oppenheim was able to rise to a position of leadership among German neurologists. He never held an official teaching post, never again held a post in any state institution, and was virtually completely deprived of the opportunity to teach within the established system. Instead of following the usual academic pathway, Oppenheim carved out his scientific career independently. His private clinic soon became an international referral center for clinical neurology, and at the same time his prolific mind and pen produced numerous publications which were read worldwide.

Unlike most of those who described variations or improvement of Babinski's cutaneous plantar reflex, Oppenheim's contributions to neurologic examination of patients with pyramidal tract lesions antedated Babinski's report. This is fitting for the protégé of the man who discovered the knee jerk. Oppenheim not only gave an early description of spasticity but also was the first to note its association with hyperreflexia.

At first Oppenheim was skeptical about the diagnostic value of the Babinski sign, but then, in 1902, he described the sign that now carries his name:

> If one draws the handle (or shaft) of a percussion hammer over the inner surface of the leg from the upper margin of the tibia downward, one sees in healthy persons either no movement at all in the foot and toes or else a plantar flexion of the toes. If the irritation is made strongly enough, distinct plantar flexion of the toes is the rule, but sometimes it is necessary to divert the attention of the patient to obviate voluntary movements. Whereas in persons with the symptom complex of spastic hemiparesis, this reflex movement of the muscles is extended to the great toe and adducts or abducts the foot.

Oppenheim had observed this sign in a number of cases of spastic paresis in which Babinski's toe phenomenon had been indistinct or doubtful, what today we might call equivocal Babinski signs. As a result, he believed and tried to convince others that his sign was more valuable than the Babinski sign.

In addition to his contributions to neurologic examination and his failure to achieve the traditional form of success, Oppenheim's career had several other parallels with that of his friend and contemporary. Like Babinski, Oppenheim was interested in the study of hysteria, especially traumatic neuroses. Oppenheim maintained that physical trauma caused neuroses only if the trauma resulted in some sort of organic disturbance in the brain, a notion that Charcot, Babinski, and others vigorously opposed. Perhaps the one similarity, which gives the best perspective of the state of neurology during the lives of Oppenheim and Babinski, was their enthusiasm in initiating neurosurgery in their respective countries. Oppenheim's diagnosis and localization resulted in the first surgical removal of a brain tumor.

In 1900 Oppenheim published the initial description of amyotonia congenita, which often is called Oppenheim's disease. In a classic paper in 1911 he first coined the term *dystonia musculorum deformans*. He also published major monographs on syphilis and encephalitis, and he was one of the first clinicians to use Paul Ehrlich's salvarsan for the treatment of neurosyphilis.

Moritz Heinrich Romberg (1795–1873)

In many respects, modern neurology began with Romberg, who has been described as the first physician to bring order and system to the study of neurologic diseases (Fig. 4). Romberg was born in Meiningen and studied medicine at the University of Berlin. Following his graduation in 1817, the 22-year-old Romberg selected his life's work and the object of all his research: the study of the diseases of the nervous system. In order to carry out these aims most efficiently, he went to Vienna, where one of his teachers was John Peter Frank (1745–1821). Frank was one of the great pioneers of public health and had written a major treatise on the pathology of the spinal cord.

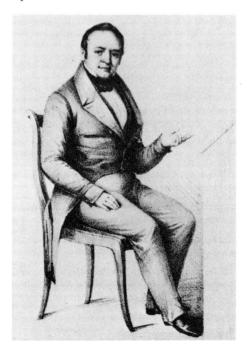

FIG. 4. Contemporary portrait of Moritz Heinrich Romberg. (From Lawrence C. McHenry, *Garrison's History of Neurology*, 1969. Courtesy of Charles C Thomas, Springfield, Ill.)

Other than his patients, two English authors were perhaps the greatest influence on Romberg. The first of these was Andrew Marshall, whose *The Morbid Anatomy of the Brain in Mania and Hydrophobia* Romberg translated into German. Marshall had been a student of William Hunter and had practiced medicine in London and lectured on surgery. In this book Marshall described the gross appearance of the brain in patients who had died of mania at the Bethlehem Hospital, and he described the gross structural abnormalities that he believed to be due to defective circulation. While the influence of Marshall's book may have been limited, the significance of the second treatise translated by Romberg, Sir Charles Bell's *Nervous System of the Human Body*, was profound. Romberg referred to Bell as "the Harvey of our century" and expressed his admiration of Bell's work in these words: "The researches of Sir Charles Bell fill me with enthusiasm, and in 1831 I translated his great work and made known to my professional brethren in Germany his investigations which will ever serve as models of scientific inquiry." Sir Charles Bell (1774–1842) worked in both Edinburgh and London as an anatomist and physiologist and performed the first experiments that demonstrated the motor function of the anterior spinal root. The distinction of being the first to clearly differentiate the sensory function of the posterior root from the motor function of the anterior root belongs to Magendie; however, in his book Bell demonstrated the motor and sensory character of the trigeminal nerve and separated it from the facial nerve, with which it had previously been confused.

As with all great clinicians, patients and their afflictions were the major influences on the work of Romberg. Romberg himself described their significance:

> I availed myself of the opportunities afforded in our large hospital, la Charité of examining all the patients labouring under cerebral disease. . . . I had extensive opportunities of examining patients during life and after death. For twenty-eight years I was physician to one of the largest unions in Berlin, in which on the average, 200 patients presented themselves annually; among them were a large number of nervous patients, most of whom I presented to my pupils in the lectures which I delivered in the University since 1834. Some of the results of these investigations have been laid down in my academical Essays.

The combined influences of his patients and his strong understanding of basic neurologic science resulted in his revolutionary *Lehrbuch de Nervenkrankheiten des Menschen*, which appeared in segments between 1840 and 1846. This textbook, which provided the first systematic approach to clinical neurology, was divided into two sections. The first dealt with diseases of sensibility or sensation, and the second dealt with disorders of motility or movement.

In the sensory section there are excellent descriptions of neuritis, causalgia, neuromas, facial neuralgia, ciliary neuralgia, sciatica, and many other conditions that we recognize today. All of these are illustrations by case histories, and full references to the literature are provided. Included in this section is a description of the nerves of muscular senses:

> Thus the healthy individual perceives motion or rest, and he becomes conscious of any variation as regards the facility of difficulty with which his muscles ac-

complish their duty. Nothing but a nerve can serve to conduct this sensation; and, if there must be a nerve to communicate the impulse of will to the muscle, there must be a second nerve which reconducts the sensation of action, and this is the nerve of muscular sense.

As Romberg was careful to point out, Bell had previously described position sense.

The section on motor disease is largely devoted to descriptions of muscular spasms, especially those concerned with breathing and talking. The space given to this topic seems inordinately large by modern standards. Later in the same volume there are excellent descriptions of chorea, tetanus, epilepsy, facial paralysis, and finally tabes dorsalis. Because of this famous description of tabes dorsalis that he presented, the sign now carries his name:

> Early in the disease we find the sense of touch and the muscular sense diminished, while the sensibility of the skin is unaltered in reference to temperature and painful impressions. The feet feel numbed in standing, walking, or lying down, and the patient has the sensation as if they were covered with a fur; the resistance of the ground is not felt as usual, its cohesion seems diminished, and the patient has a sensation as if the sole of his foot were in contact with wool, soft sand, or a bladder filled with water. The rider no longer feels the resistance of the stirrup, and has the strap put up a hole or two. The gait begins to be insecure, and the patient attempts to improve it by making a greater effort of the will; as he does not feel the tread to be firm, he puts down his heels with greater force. From the commencement of the disease the individual keeps his eyes on his feet to prevent his movements from becoming still more unsteady. If he is ordered to close his eyes while in the erect posture, he at once commences to totter and swing from side to side; the insecurity of his gait also exhibits itself in the dark. It is now ten years since I pointed out this pathognomonic sign, and it is a symptom which I have not observed in other paralyses, nor in uncomplicated amaurosis; since then I have found it in a considerable number of patients, from far and near, who have applied for my advice; in no case have I found it wanting. Some patients mention the circumstance without being asked about it; one gentleman, a foreigner, whose eyesight was unimpaired, told me that he was at present unable to wash himself in his dark bedroom while standing; and that if he wished to keep his balance he was obliged to have a light while performing his toilet. Another, whose business rendered it necessary for him to go out at six o'clock in the morning, complained that he required one to support him in the house and out of doors, but that he could dispense with assistance in full daylight.

He also recorded the pain that often plagues these patients:

> Painful sensations of different kinds almost invariably accompany the affection; the most common is a sense of constriction, which proceeds from the dorsal or lumbar vertebrae, encircles the trunk like a hoop, and not unfrequently renders breathing laborious. Several of my patients have described this sensation as particularly troublesome during sleep, causing them suddenly to start up and scream out.

Romberg even observed some of the pupillary changes that accompany tabes:

> Even when the optic nerve was not implicated, I have repeatedly found a change in the pupils of one or both eyes, consisting in a contraction with loss of motion, which in one case, that of a man aged 45, attained to such a height that the pupils were reduced to the size of a pin's head.

Although this was the first organized description of this disease and of the Romberg sign, Romberg never recognized the relationship between tabes dorsalis and syphilis.

Romberg gained great fame as a clinical neurologist, teacher, and neuropathologist. In 1838 he was appointed Professor Extraordinaire for pathology, and in 1840 he became director of the university hospital. His textbook went through three editions and numerous translations and had a profound influence on the subsequent development of clinical neurology.

The words of his preface to the second edition of his Lehrbuch summarized his view of neurology:

> The study of nervous diseases which some persons have refused to acknowledge as anything but the manifestations of other morbid processes, has been declared a fruitless research, and in some schools has been almost interdicted. . . . To guard against greater debasement, we must enter anew upon the path which the mastermind of Charles Bell, the Harvey of our century, has opened to us.
>
> Let our guide be the analysis of observations, not the cavilling spirit which even attacks the solid basis of physiological laws, such as the law of eccentrical phenomena, or the law of prohibiting one nerve from acting for another, but that purifying criticism which lays bare defects, and mercilessly eradicates fallacies and untruths.

Guillaume Benjamin Amand Duchenne (1806–1875)

While Romberg, with his systematic approach grounded in thorough knowledge of neuroanatomy and neuropathology, brought order to German neurology, G. B. A. Duchenne, without benefit of any such background, initiated French neurology. It is said that Duchenne (Fig. 5) found French neurology as "a sprawling infant of unknown parentage which he succored to a lusty youth." Duchenne was born in the seaport town of Boulogne-sur-Mer. For many generations his ancestors had been fishermen, sea captains, and traders. His father had been awarded the Croix de la Legion d'Honneur in 1804 by order of Napoleon Bonaparte as a result of his actions as a ship's captain in the war between France and England. At age 19, Duchenne went to study medicine at the University of Paris, then the greatest medical school in the world, boasting such teachers as Cruveilhier, Dupuytren, and Laennec. He graduated in 1831 and returned to Boulogne-sur-Mer to settle down as a general practitioner. He gave little if any thought to the study of neurologic diseases. His life was soon shattered by the death of his wife. She died giving birth to their son, and her sudden death caused what we would now call a prolonged depression, during which he gave up medicine, spending much of his time just sitting on the lonely waterfront. This barren period lasted 9 years. During this time he became alienated from his friends and family, including his son. Finally he returned to Paris.

In Paris he had no hospital appointment. At first he had no powerful friends in the medical world. However, he did have a goal, which he pursued with all his boundless energy. His goal was to understand the functioning of human muscles

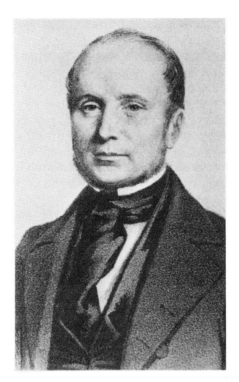

FIG. 5. Portrait of Guillaume Benjamin Amand Duchenne. (From Webb Haymaker, *The Founders of Neurology*, 1953. Courtesy of Charles C Thomas, Springfield, Ill.)

and the diseases that alter their functioning. In order to achieve this goal, Duchenne, who now called himself Duchenne de Boulogne to avoid being confused with Duchenne de Paris, studied the effects of faradic current on the muscular activity of patients. He tirelessly went from hospital to hospital talking to and examining patient after patient. Once a patient interested him, he would even follow the patient to the patient's home. At first he was considered a strange interloper, but Duchenne de Boulogne soon gained a reputation as an honest, hard-working clinical observer who was both skillful and kind-hearted. He was not well read in neurologic science. Through most of his productive life, for instance, he was ignorant of the work of Romberg. He was entirely self-taught in neurology, using his patients and his examinations of them as his only textbook. As his reputation increased, this iconoclast began to make friends within the medical establishment. Two of these friends, Trousseau and Charcot, played major roles in helping Duchenne, who was absent-minded and relatively inarticulate, to publish his findings.

Because his major interest was in observing the effects of electrical stimulation on individual muscles, it was natural that his major contributions were in the realm of disorders of mobility. His first major book, *De L'Electrisation Localisée et de son Application à la Pathologie et à la Therapeutique*, came out in 1855. It led to a great deal of interest in faradic stimulation as a therapeutic modality (Fig. 6). In the long run, of course, electrotherapy proved to be of little value. The third edition, which appeared in 1872, is of more interest today because of its analysis of facial expression and a complete review of the functioning of individual muscles.

Duchenne's lasting contributions to the development of neurology include his clinical descriptions of four major disorders of motility: progressive spinal muscular atrophy; pseudohypertrophic muscular dystrophy; bulbar palsy, which he called glossolabio-laryngeal paralysis; poliomyelitis. Not a bad list of accomplishments for a man without training.

In 1848, Duchenne described a patient with progressive muscular atrophy beginning distally in the arms and slowly spreading proximally and eventually involving the trunk and legs. Accounts of this patient and other patients of Duchenne were published by François Amilcar Aran, who was then physician to the Hôpital Saint Antoine. Aran, in his paper, clearly acknowledged Duchenne's pivotal contribution: "I owe a thousand thanks to my friend Duchenne (of Boulogne) who freely put at my disposal all his material, and without officious intervention." It is fitting that primary muscular atrophy is often called Aran-Duchenne disease; for

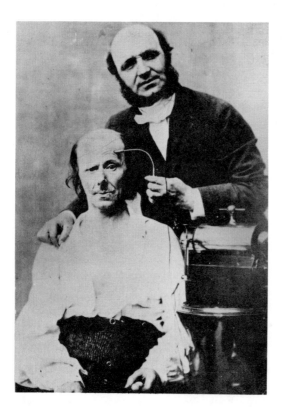

FIG. 6. Duchenne de Boulogne demonstrating contracting of the frontalis muscle following application of faradic current. (From Lawrence C. McHenry, *Garrison's History of Neurology*, 1969. Courtesy of Charles C Thomas, Springfield, Ill.)

although the honor for isolating this disorder belongs to Duchenne, without Aran this knowledge might never have been disseminated.

Some 8 years after Duchenne's death, the New Sydenham Society published his contributions on progressive spinal muscular atrophy, translated, edited, and condensed by G. V. Poore:

> Progressive muscular atrophy attacks the upper limb, and destroys its muscles in an irregular fashion. It begins in such cases by attacking one after another the muscles of the thenar eminence, spreading from the superficial to the deep layer. As the abductor pollicis is wasted, its absence is marked by a depression, and by the attitude, during repose, of the first metacarpal bone, which lies too close to the second. . . . Depressions of the hypothenar eminence and interosseal spaces next announce the atrophy of the muscles of those regions. The triceps extensor cubiti is the last of the muscles of the upper limb to become affected. . . . The atrophy equally invades the lower limbs, but only when the muscles of the upper limbs and trunk are in great part destroyed.

In these patients Duchenne studied the pathologic findings in the atrophic muscles and described the atrophy of the large cells of the anterior horn of the spinal cord. However, he was never certain whether the cord lesions were primary or secondary. It was Charcot who later solved this problem.

Armed with his newly won understanding of a direct relationship between anterior horn cell atrophy and muscle atrophy, it should not surprise us that Duchenne predicted that lesions of the bulbar motor nuclei would be found in patients whom he described with progressive bulbar palsy. Such brilliant clinico-pathologic predictions have occurred only rarely in the history of neurology. In following his patients with disease that produced atrophy, Duchenne was also the first to demonstrate involvement of the anterior horn in poliomyelitis.

The contribution for which he is best remembered is his description of pseudo-hypertrophic muscular dystrophy published in 1868.

> The disease I will describe is characterized principally by: (1) weakness of movements, usually settling at first in the muscles of the lower extremities and the lumbar spine, then spreading to the upper extremities at the terminal stage and worsening at the same time until movement is abolished; (2) increase in volume either (ordinarily) in several of the paralyzed muscles or (exceptionally) in nearly all the paralyzed muscles; (3) hyperplasia of the interstitial connective tissue of the paralyzed muscles, with an abundant production of fibrous tissue or of fatty vesicles in the more advanced stage.
>
> I propose to call this disease pseudohypertrophic muscular paralysis after its principal objective clinical signs or myosclerotic paralysis after its peripheral anatomic characteristics. These terms will be justified by studying the symptomatology and the pathologic anatomy in the living during the course of the disease. I prefer the first of these terms.

These articles included illustrations of patients and of the pathology in the musculature. The latter were derived from percutaneous muscle biopsy. This technique was developed by Duchenne and was the first that allowed for safe evaluation of

F. 24. F. 25. F. 26. F. 27.

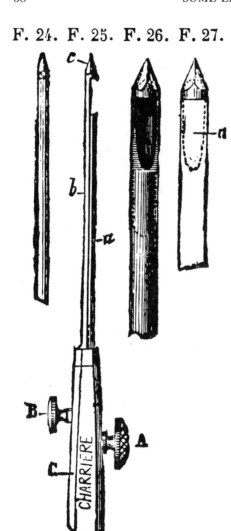

FIG. 7. Duchenne de Boulogne's original muscle biopsy harpoon.

muscle pathology during the life of the patient. The biopsy apparatus, which Gower called Duchenne's "histological harpoon," is shown in Fig. 7.

In 1862 Duchenne's son joined him in Paris and began the study of neurology under his tutelage. This was a happy time for Duchenne. He still had no hospital appointment in Paris, no academic chair, no official teaching position. Neither the Academie de Medecine nor the Institut de France honored him. But his reputation was growing worldwide. He was elected to corresponding memberships in academic medical societies in Rome, Madrid, Stockholm, Geneva, Leipzig, and even Saint Petersburg. He had the support of his friends, especially Charcot, who always acknowledged his debt to Duchenne and was always ready to help Duchenne make his discoveries known. Duchenne devoted himself to his son's academic development, but in 1871 his son died of typhoid fever. Duchenne, who had taken 9 years to recover from the death of his wife, never rebounded from the death of his son. He died 4 years later of a cerebral hemorrhage.

One other contribution of Duchenne is often overlooked. He was one of the first physicians to use photography to preserve and present microscopic findings.

Should we really honor such men as Duchenne eponymously, or should we follow the advice of Sir William Gowers (Gowers' sign):

> There are very few observations in medicine regarding which it is not obvious that they would speedily have been made by someone other than the actual observer; that is very much of an accident that they were made by certain individuals. Scientific nomenclature should be itself scientific, not founded upon accidents. However anxious we may be to honor individuals, we have no right to do so at the expense of the convenience of all future generations of learners.

Charcot himself may have given the best answer. In one of his *Leçons de Mardi* he recorded his discussion of a case of Duchenne's pseudohypertrophic muscular dystrophy and asked these questions:

> How is it that one fine morning Duchenne discovered a disease that probably existed in the time of Hippocrates?.... Why do we perceive things so late, so poorly, with such difficulty! Why do we have to go over the same set of symptoms twenty times before we understand it? Why does the first statement of what seems a new fact always leave us cold?

He then went on to answer them:

> Because our minds have to take in something that deranges our original set of ideas, but we are all of us like that in this miserable world.

Only few clinicians are able to abstract observations that identify a "new" disease or change how we think about an "old" disease. Such men should not be forgotten.

Addendum: Hoffmann's Sign

The reflex known as Hoffmann's sign is not without interest from the historical point of view, since it shows that there may exist considerable confusion even about recent medical discoveries. Today each neurological and even each complete physical examination includes the test for this sign, because its presence is considered to be an excellent sign of hyperreflexia, similar to the Babinski phenomenon.

In spite of its general usefulness and fame, nothing had appeared in the literature to suggest who Hoffmann was, and why his name was attached to this sign.

O. Blenheim (1936)

The sign associated with the name of Johann Hoffmann (1857–1919) ranks with those of Babinski and Romberg as one of the most widely used and accepted of all eponyms. Its history differs greatly from the histories of almost all other famous signs in that its discoverer never published a description of it.

Hoffmann, like Oppenheim, was a student of Wilhelm Heinrich Erb (1840–1921), whose many contributions to neurology included his discovery of the knee jerk:

> For quite some time I have observed in healthy persons, but particularly in patients with lesions of the spinal cord, well developed reflexes in the quadriceps femoris which are readily and promptly elicited and which I deem worthy of some attention and practical evaluation. They can be produced by slight tapping of the tendon of the quadriceps above as well as below the patella, particularly from the region of the patellar ligament. These reflexes indicate an intimate and close reflex relationship between this tendon and the associated muscles.
>
> I do not believe that this observation is entirely new to my colleagues in neurology; it is probable that the majority are familiar with this manifestation. Nevertheless, the literature is almost completely silent about this and similar facts, which certainly are not without interest. Quite recently I have gone over a large volume of the literature on the physiology and pathology of the spinal cord and I have found no unequivocal and adequate reports about it, unless the statements in question were just the ones that escaped me.
>
> For this reason I believe that a brief mention of these tendon reflexes should be permissible, especially because they have proved to be a frequent and readily demonstrable manifestation which certainly must have some diagnostic importance that should not be underestimated; because they occur moreover, as a rule, with greater clearness and significance than do the skin reflexes, with which the tendon reflexes are not always in parallel, and finally because I have observed them in many tendons in addition to the quadriceps.

Hoffmann succeeded Erb as professor of neurology at Heidelberg, and his name is also associated with spinal muscular atrophy in children, which he described in 1891.

He apparently hit upon his sign prior to 1904 and demonstrated it in his lectures and clinics, but its first description in the literature was by Hoffmann's student Hans Curschmann in 1911. Curschmann had been Hoffmann's assistant from 1901 to 1904 and must have learned the sign then. In his paper he named the reflex the Hoffmann sign.

Two other authors contributed to this sign. In 1913, Tromner, a neurologist from Hamburg who was unaware of the Hoffmann-Curschmann paper, described virtually the same sign, and in 1908 Jakobsohn described a very similar sign that he accomplished without snapping the fingernail.

NOTES

There is no full-scale English-language biography of any of the neurologists discussed here. The most complete biographical sketch of Joseph Babinski is by Pearce Bailey (*World Neurology* 2:134–140, 1962). John Fulton's appreciation of Babinski's career appeared in the *Journal of Nervous and Mental Diseases* (77:121–131, 1933), and his obituary was published in *Archives of Neurology and Psychiatry* (29:168–174, 1933). George Guillain's *J. M. Charcot*, translated by Pearce Bailey (1959, Hoeber), gives details of neurology and medicine in Paris during the early part of Babinski's career. This source also gives valuable information about Duchenne. There are brief biographical sketches of Babinski, Oppenheim, Romberg, and Duchenne de Boulogne in *The Founders of Neurology*, edited by W. Haymaker and F. Schiller (1953, Charles C Thomas). This and L. C. McHenry's revised edition of *Garrison's History of Neurology* (1969, Charles C Thomas) are recommended to anyone who wants more information on the individuals who molded modern neurology.

Romberg's textbook was translated by E. H. Sieveking and published by the New Sydenham Society of London in 1853. The same society published its edited collection of Duchenne's papers in 1883.

A Mithridate for Paracelsus

Mithridates, he died old.

A. E. Houseman, *A Shropshire Lad*

Paracelsus, he died young.

A Mithridate for Paracelsus

Paracelsus, who lived from 1493 to 1541, is generally considered to have been the most original medical thinker of the sixteenth century and the greatest single reformer of Renaissance medicine. As such, he is often called the Luther of medicine. During his lifetime his reputation and contributions provoked heated and even violent debate. For every admirer who compared him to Martin Luther, there was at least one detractor who regarded him as a dangerous heretic who should be burned at the stake. This controversy lasts to this day.

Benjamin Gordon, in his book *Medieval and Renaissance Medicine*, attributed to Paracelsus the true temperament of a practical physician who learned more from his daily contacts with patients than from any of the books he had studied. It was his practice to instruct his students at the bedside of a sick patient rather than in the lecture halls of the universities. The secret of his success was his appeal to the common people. He lectured and wrote in German, not in Latin. Latin was the language of instruction throughout Europe, and it was used by all of the university professors who were his contemporaries. These two departures from standard teaching practices (bedside instruction of students and instruction in the vernacular) have today become cornerstones of medical education. In the sixteenth century they were radical departures that bordered on heresy.

These were not his only revolutionary ideas. He was one of the first to break away from the orthodox schools of Galen and Avicenna. The writings of these two authorities had long dominated European medical thought. Physicians treated their books as reverently as the church treated the works of the Apostles. Paracelsus did not. He applied to medical problems the same kind of independent thought that Luther employed in religion and Galileo in astronomy. Paracelsus, rather than relying totally on authorities, used his own observations and experiences. "The human mind," according to Paracelsus, "knows nothing of the nature of things from the inward meditations. . . . That which his eyes see and his hands touch, that is his teacher. . . . Science is a search for God in his creation and medicine is God's gift to man."

Even modern medical historians often are ambivalent in their views of Paracelsus. Garrison, for instance, clearly recognized his contribution, but still compared Paracelsus to the "roarers" of Elizabethan comedy and stated that Paracelsus often tried to bully and browbeat his readers into accepting his views. His writings, according to Garrison, are a curious mixture of fact, fustian, and swagger, set off by many successful guesses at truth and some remarkable intuitions, and his humorous sallies, if he intended them as such, usually drift from the obscene into the incomprehensible.

The controversy that surrounds Paracelsus begins with his name and ends with his death. All agree that he was born in Einsiedeln, Switzerland, near Zurich, in 1493. Various sources disagree on his original name and also on the meaning of his assumed name Paracelsus. His name has been recorded as Theophrastus Bombastus von Hohenheim, Aureolus Theophrastus Bombastus von Hohenheim, Philippus Theophrastus Aurealus Paracelsus Bambas von Hohenheim, and other variants. It has been suggested either that the English word *bombast* is derived from the writing style of Paracelsus or, at worst, that both his name and the English word come from a single source which through some quirk, also describes Paracelsus' manner of communication. Alas, the truth is more prosaic. The word *bombax* was widely used in the Middle Ages as the popular name for cotton, apparently derived from the Greek and later Latin word for silk. By the sixteenth century the English word *bombast* was used to describe cotton wool used as padding or stuffing in clothes. Anyone wearing such clothes would, of course, present a false image of his physique, would be falsely inflated. Thus, over the years, the word *bombast* acquired a metaphorical meaning of inflated language. This derivation had nothing to do with Paracelsus, whose family name also referred back to the material meaning of the word. The allegorical meaning now attached to the word *bombast* did not reach back from England to Germanic areas of Europe until at least a century after his family had taken the name *Bombastus*. In later life he assumed the name Paracelsus, by which he is now known. It is unclear what this name signified to Theophrastus Bombastus von Hohenheim. Some authorities maintain that by taking this name he was proclaiming his equality with Celsus. This may be possible, but Paracelsus in his own writing never even mentioned Celsus and certainly did not proclaim Celsus to have been an authority worthy of being equaled. In fact, it is not entirely clear that Paracelsus had even heard of or read Celsus. Celsus was an ancient authority figure who was considered an expert in medicine without even having been a physician, an unlikely inspiration for Paracelsus. Others think the name was merely an attempt to Latinize the German name Hohenheim, a popular practice in his day. Others believe that the name Paracelsus is simply the Latin phrase *para celsus*, meaning equal to the eminent or very eminent.

Paracelsus (Fig. 1) was the son of a learned physician named Wilhelm Bombast von Hohenheim, who was a graduate of Tübingen and was in charge of the hospital attached to the convent of Einsiedeln. When Theophrastus, as he was then known, was 9 years old, his father was appointed town physician at Villach in Corinthia. There young Theophrastus began the study of medicine with his father and probably attended a school of mines, where he developed a lifelong interest in metals, mining, and the diseases of miners.

His formal education began at the University of Basel, but he soon left Basel for Würzburg to study with Trithemus, who was a renowned alchemist. For a 10-year period from 1517 to 1526 he traveled over much of Europe gathering knowledge from both orthodox and unorthodox sources. His early travels carried him to universities and medical centers in Vienna, Cologne, Paris, Montpellier, and then Italy. While studying in Italy, he apparently received the degree of doctor of medicine from the University of Ferrara. From Italy he went to Spain, England, and Holland, where he served as a surgeon in the Dutch army. In 1518 he was a surgeon in the Danish army besieging Stockholm. Later he traveled to Pomerania, Lithuania,

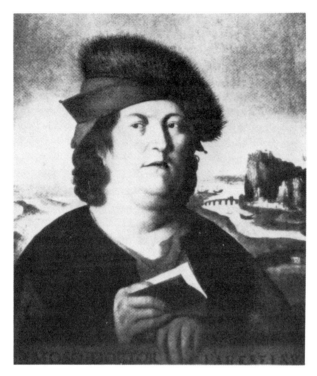

FIG. 1. Portrait of Paracelsus at age 24, by Scorel, painted in 1517 and now in the Louvre. (From Ralph H. Major, *A History of Medicine*, 1954. Courtesy of Charles C Thomas, Springfield, Ill.)

Poland, Russia, Hungary, Wallachia, Transylvania, Dalmatia, and Venice, where he served in the Venetian armies. Throughout his wandering he tirelessly collected information from every possible source, including barbers, executioners, bathkeepers, gypsies, midwives, and fortune-tellers. He learned a great deal from these sources about the practice of medicine, and he acquired an unusual knowledge of folk medicine and a permanent taste for low company. After some time in Venice, which was then the gateway to the Levant, Paracelsus decided to continue his studies in the East. He traveled to Egypt and Constantinople, which was already under Turkish control. In these centers of Islamic learning he continued his study of alchemy and Eastern mysticism. Back in the West he rejoined the Venetian army, which was then fighting Charles V. Finally, after 9 years of wandering, Paracelsus returned to Strassburg, hoping to settle there as a surgeon. At this point, fate, in the guise of a grateful patient, played a major role in shaping his career.

Johann Froben or Frobenius, a famous Renaissance humanist, printer, and publisher, was suffering from a severe, persistent leg infection. The leading surgeons of Basel had all advocated amputation in order to save Froben's life. Froben was unhappy with this choice. He had heard of the clinical prowess of Paracelsus and asked him to come to Basel. Paracelsus came to Basel and undertook Froben's medical care. Although his exact treatment regimen is unknown, Paracelsus saved both Froben's leg and his life. In gratitude, Froben managed to get the city council to appoint Paracelsus to the office of municipal physician and professor at the University of Basel. The faculty was outraged. Paracelsus was not an academic scholar. In the eyes of the established faculty his credentials were questionable and his philosophies were outrageous. As Paracelsus himself said, "I pleased no one, except the sick whom I healed." If his reputation antagonized the faculty, Paracelsus himself scandalized them. He taught students in their own language, not in Latin. Worse yet, he taught them at the bedside, using real patients, not ancient textbooks. His attitude toward his fellow faculty members did not help gain their acceptance, not that his words had that goal in mind:

> All the universities have less experience than my beard. The down on my neck is more learned than my antagonists. You must follow my footsteps. I shall not go in yours. Not one of your professors will find a cover so well hidden that the dogs will come and lift them by the legs and defile them. I shall become a monarch, mine will be the monarchy which I shall rule to make you gird up your loins.

He went so far as to publicly burn copies of the writings of Avicenna and Galen in the students' St. John's Day bonfire.

His success in curing Frobenius not only brought him to Basel but also gave him access to Frobenius's printing press. Paracelsus lost no time in taking full advantage of this position. In pamphlet after pamphlet he continued his attack on the medical establishment.

> Very few physicians have exact knowledge of disease and the causes but my books are not like those of other physicians copying Hippocrates and Galen. I have composed them on the basis of experiments which are the greatest masters of everything, and with indefatigable labor. If any of you feel the desire to penetrate the divine secrets of medicine and feel like acquiring the medical art in the shortest time come to me at Basel and you will find much more than I can promise you with my words.

None of this won him any friends, and finally he had to flee Basel in the dark of night, fearing for his life. Afraid that he would be poisoned, he took a mithridate of his own concoction. His wandering continued until 1540, when he was finally offered asylum by the bishop of Salzburg. He spent his remaining few days in Salzburg in relative quiet and died on September 24, 1541, at the age of 48, of natural causes (Fig. 2). Some claim that this natural cause was cancer. Others blame a wound received in a tavern brawl, a consequence of a drunken debauch of some days' duration. Some claim that his death resulted from having been thrown down from a high place by agents of either physicians or apothecaries, or that having run out of mithridate he finally succumbed to poison administered by one of the groups he had harassed for so many years.

Paracelsus reformed the practice of medicine in many ways. His approach was his own, not that of the traditional authorities. He rejected ancient, often pagan, philosophies and systems and substituted his own. He believed that the four pillars of medicine were philosophy, astrology, alchemy, and virtue. His own philosophy

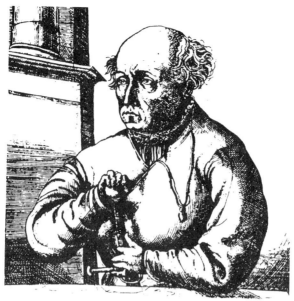

FIG. 2. An engraving of Paracelsus at the age of 47, the year before his untimely death, by Augustin Hirshvogel. (From Ralph H. Major, *A History of Medicine*, 1954. Courtesy of Charles C Thomas, Springfield, Ill.)

was essentially mystical, and it appears to us to be cloudy at best and of little real concern. His view of astrology was based on ancient beliefs concerning the relationship between the universe and man. According to this theory, Jupiter ruled the liver, Mars the gallbladder, the moon the brain, the sun the heart, Saturn the spleen, Mercury the lungs, and Venus the kidneys. The same types of influences were exerted by various metals. Gold corresponded to the sun, silver to the moon, lead to Saturn, mercury to Mercury, copper to Venus, tin to Jupiter, iron to Mars. There were similar correspondences in regard to plants. In the field of alchemy, Paracelsus asserted that each element (fire, earth, water, air) was divisible into three parts: salt, sulfur, and mercury. Virtue, the fourth pillar of medicine, consisted of obedience to the will of God, as revealed through the workings of nature and the teachings of Christ.

In discussing the causes of diseases, Paracelsus rejected the traditional view that health depended on a proper balance of the four humors: phlegm, blood, yellow bile, and black bile. In place of this humoral theory, he developed his own theory of five entities or active principles: the *ens astrale*, the *ens veneni*, the *ens naturale*, the *ens spirituale*, and the *ens dei*. The *ens astrale* was the influence of the stars, *ens veneni* the influence of other persons, *ens naturale* the influence of oneself, *ens spirituale* the influence of the spirit, and *ens dei* the will of God. Although this was broader than the humoral theory, this conceptualization was also more philosophical than scientific.

What were the achievements of this revolutionary? His major contributions related more to his personality and his style than to any great scientific advances. His challenging of ancient authority by the use of clinical observation and by the use of modern language was long overdue, but these innovations gained acceptance only slowly. His major reformation had to do with therapeutics. In many respects he was the predecessor and initiator of chemical pharmacology and therapeutics. He was one of the first to advocate the use of chemical agents for treatment of specific diseases.

Paracelsus believed that all medicines were the creation of God. However, God did not prepare them in such a manner that they were ready for human administration. God had placed the active ingredients or principles within a slag, hiding them among inactive impurities. It was the job of the physician to remove the active principles from the slag. Paracelsus believed that all things had been created in an impure form, and it remained for physicians to convert them into pure or ultimate forms through alchemy, which was the art of separating the useful from the useless.

He firmly believed that nature was sufficient for the cure of most diseases and that medicine had to intervene only when the internal physician, the patient himself, became exhausted or incapable of responding. Then and only then should the physician introduce some remedy that would be antagonistic to the disease process. Using this approach, Paracelsus taught his followers to carry out therapeutic experiments, not to rely blindly on traditional authority. This one philosophically muddled but simple approach provided the cornerstone for the development of successful therapeutic agents, and it is perhaps his major contribution to the practice of medicine.

The followers of Paracelsus were clearly distinguishable from the members of the Galenic school by their use of chemical agents in the practice of medicine. Paracelsus and his followers discovered a number of drugs that proved to be of value. Paracelsus himself introduced mineral baths and was one of the first to analyze them. Through Paracelsus, opium, laudanum, mercury, lead, sulfur, iron, arsenic, copper sulfate, and potassium sulfate became accepted as part of the pharmacopoeia. Paracelsus also contributed to the advancement of chemistry. He distinguished alum from ferrous sulfate, and he demonstrated the iron content of water by use of gallic acid. He popularized new forms of medical preparations such as extracts and tinctures. Some have claimed that Paracelsus is also the father of anesthesia. Unquestionably he did describe the anesthetic action of sulfuric ether on chickens, and he stated that it "quiets all suffering without any harm, and relieves all pain." Being a product of his time, he relied on the so-called doctrine of signatures in his selection of therapeutic agents. This doctrine held that God created plants in forms that suggested the organs on which they would act. According to this theory, an infusion of specula pennara should be given for diseases of the breast, because the shape of the plant resembles that of the breasts. In the same way, topaz alandine and other yellow substances should be beneficial in the treatment of jaundice. Furthermore, yellow substances should be beneficial in heart disease, because yellow is the color of the sun, which rules the heart.

Paracelsus had a great interest in syphilis, which had just appeared in Europe and was spreading at an epidemic rate. He divided syphilis into local and general, primary and secondary. In his writings he described the inheritance of syphilis, as well as its numerous forms and its influence on the courses of other diseases. Paracelsus concocted a great number of mercurial preparations, following alchemy formulas, that he then used for the treatment of syphilis. He erroneously regarded gonorrhea as an initial stage of syphilis, but he was correct in ascribing the cause, or at least the cause of the dissemination of this epidemic, to sexual contact.

The other major epidemic of his day was the dancing mania. This, more than syphilis, was a true product of its age. Groups of sufferers with an irresistible urge to dance wandered over much of Europe, spreading the contagion wherever they went. Like syphilis, this was a new disease. In contrast to the base origin of syphilis, most contemporaries believed that the dancing mania had a supranatural origin and that the victims of this scourge could be saved only by the intervention of Saint Vitus, whose name became associated with the contagion (Fig. 3). Paracelsus became particularly interested in this phenomenon, and he loudly protested against this or any other disease being attributed to the devil or being named after a saint. Despite his customary rejection of ancient authorities, he accepted the rational reasoning of Hippocrates and insisted that all diseases could be ascribed to natural causes. He totally rejected the notion that Saint Vitus could intervene to cure this affliction. Rather than invoking superhuman forces, Paracelsus devised his own harsh but effective treatment for the dancing mania. He treated the victims of this apparent form of mass hysteria with such heroic measures as immersion in cold water, fasting, and solitary confinement. As his therapeutic approach gained ac-

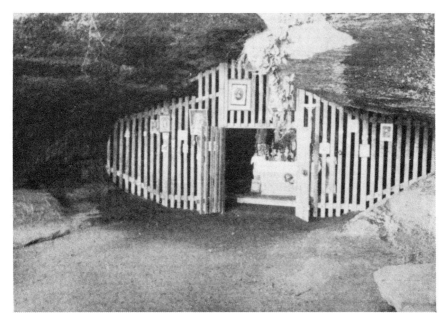

FIG. 3. Chapel of Saint Vitus near Saverne (Zabern), Alsace, France. (From Ralph H. Major, *A History of Medicine*, 1954. Courtesy of Charles C Thomas, Springfield, Ill.)

ceptance, the outbreaks of the dancing mania began to subside. Whether the cure itself or the threat of it effected the cessation of these peculiar dances is a question that is still unanswered.

Paracelsus made other clinical contributions to medicine. He was the first to recognize the close relationship between endemic goiter and cretinism. His monograph on *Diseases that Deprive Man of His Reason* is a classic in the history of psychiatry and one of the first clear declarations that such afflictions are diseases and not evidence of supranatural forces.

Another of his books, *On Miners Diseases*, written in 1524, is one of the first works ever written on occupational medicine. In it he described the pulmonary and other diseases of miners, smelter workers, and metallurgists. He not only discussed etiology, pathogenesis, diagnosis, and therapy for these diseases but also discussed their prevention. His contributions in this area had a definite influence on the development of occupational and preventive medicine.

Paracelsus always mixed his medical knowledge with alchemy, magic, and what we would call showmanship. However, his treatments were always aimed at the cause of an illness, not its symptoms. He claimed to have distilled a quintessence of metals that possessed universal health-giving properties. He fostered the belief that this "universal arcanum," which was capable of curing all diseases, was hidden in the handle of a large sword that he always carried with him. He also prepared a mithridate that he took to prevent his enemies from poisoning him. His fear that his enemies might want to poison him probably was not merely paranoia on his part. This small, slight man with an unruly fringe of hair framing a large bald skull set with blazing eyes had fiercely attacked the errors and follies of medieval physicians and apothecaries, two groups with sufficient knowledge and sufficient reason to want to poison this troublemaker. In an attempt to prevent this, each day he took a mithridate. The mithridate was a time-honored universal antidote, a complex formula that had been handed down from the ancients. Ancient history recorded many Mithridates. Who was the Mithridates who invented this antidote and who himself died old?

Mithridates VI, the inventor of the universal antidote, was not an alchemist but king of the petty kingdom of Pontus in Asia Minor (Fig. 4). He was the sixth and last king of that name to reign in Pontus, and during his lifetime he fought three major wars with Rome.

Today Asia Minor is a politically unified peninsula constituting much of the modern state of Turkey. It is bounded on the north by the Black Sea, on the west by the Aegean, and on the south by the Mediterranean. But political unity was not the usual condition in ancient Asia Minor. Most of Asia Minor is a high plateau, hot and dry in summer and bitterly cold in winter. To the north, where the plateau descends to the Pontic or Black Sea, there are ranges of mountains and wooded hills, among which are fertile valleys and plains, rivers and lakes. It is a peculiarity of these mountain ranges and of their rivers and valleys that most of them run parallel to the coast, so that the rivers are navigable for only a short distance from the sea. The Roman historian Strabo was born in Amasia, the capital of the early

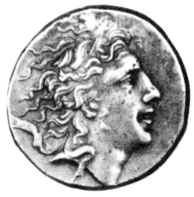

FIG. 4. Tetradrachma of Mithridates VI. Obverse shows head of Mithridates with flowing hair. Reverse shows a stag feeding. ΓΚΕ to right signifies year 223 of Pontic era, which corresponds to 74 B.C.E. Legend translates "of King Mithridates, the noble born."

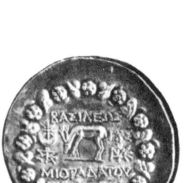

Pontic kings, which is located on one of these rivers. He has left us with a vivid, if not lyrical, description of his homeland:

> The plain is always moist and covered with grass and can support herds of cattle and horses alike and admits of the sowing of millet seed and sorghum seeds in great, or rather unlimited quantities. Indeed their plenty of water offsets any drought, so that no famine comes down on these people, never once, and the country along the mountain yields so much fruit, apples and nuts, that those who go out to the forest at any time in the year get an abundant supply, and numerous also are the catches of wild animals, because of the good yield of food.

Agriculture was not the only wealth of Pontus; minerals also played an important role in its history and economy. Large sources of copper, silver, and, most important, easily worked iron ore were available. In fact, ancient sources attribute the initial discovery of iron to the tribes of this region. In remote antiquity these people had begun to hammer the lumps of native copper lying about on the plateau. First the copper was hammered into sheets and then later into weapons and utensils.

When the supply of easily worked copper nuggets ran out, they started melting the copper out of the rocks in which they found copper ore. Later, tin was added to the copper in order to produce much harder bronze. Finally, some unknown genius began experimenting with the melting of other darker ores and discovered iron, the greatest source of arms and armament.

The history of the Mithridates kings of Pontus begins like the biblical story of David and Jonathan. The father of Mithridates I was a Persian nobleman. Pontus, like the rest of the Persian Empire, had become part of the empire of Alexander the Great. Following the death of Alexander (323 B.C.E.), his generals (the Successors of Alexander) divided the empire and began a long series of internecine wars for control of the Hellenistic world. The former comrades who now fought each other included Antigonus, who controlled Asia Minor, Seleucus, who began as governor of Babylonia, and Ptolemy, who established himself in Egypt. Mithridates I, with his son, was allied with Antigonus Gonatas, the one-eyed. Antigonus, never a trusting soul, became suspicious of both Mithridates I and his son and decided to put them to death. But meanwhile, Antigonus's son Demetrius and the young Mithridates had become close friends, and Demetrius gave his friend warning of his father's plan, much as Jonathan had warned David. Both Mithridates I and his son fled, but in different directions. The father was caught and killed, but the young Mithridates escaped. Other than this story, little is known of the vicissitudes of the early kings of Pontus, most of whom were named Mithridates. Pontus did not achieve anything like political independence for at least another 100 years, and it did not begin to issue its own coins, a true measure of independence, until well into the reign of Mithridates III (c. 220–185 B.C.E.).

Mithridates VI Eupator (the Great) reigned from 120 to 63 B.C.E. At the age of 11 his father's death left him heir to the throne, but his mother Laodice took power as regent. It soon became apparent that Laodice liked being regent and would never relinquish her power. Friends who feared for the boy's life hid him in the mountains. There he grew into a strong, skillful, and resourceful warrior and leader, with all of his mother's passion for power. After 7 years of hiding in the hinterland with the help of friends (or, perhaps more accurately, his mother's enemies), he took the capital, imprisoned his mother, killed his younger brother, and became king.

Mithridates VI built an enormous reputation for courage and athletic prowess. He was a gargantuan eater and drinker. He was fluent in several languages and was a warm friend to Greek men of letters. He lived and ruled as an oriental monarch. He was generous to his friends and intimates, but he was also suspicious, cruel, and murderous. Toward the end of his career he ordered the killing of the 500 women of his harem to prevent them falling into the hands of his enemies. During a time when Rome was beset by internal strife, he waged three long wars against Rome before finally being defeated by Pompey the Great in 63 B.C.E. He eventually took his own life. Only Hannibal had been as formidable an enemy of Rome.

Plutarch told how the news of the death of "Rome's ancient and inveterate enemy" was received by Pompey's army: "Pompey . . . told them the news of Mithridates' death, how he had put an end to his life upon the revolt of his son Pharnaces. Upon this news the whole army, expressing their joy, as was to be expected, fell to sacrificing to the gods, and feasting as if in the person of Mithridates alone there had died many thousands of their enemies."

The fame of Mithridates VI rests not only on his ability to wage three prolonged wars against Rome but also on his interest in poisons and antidotes. It is easy to see how this interest began. While his mother was regent he realized that she enjoyed power and would not easily relinquish it when he reached his majority. This was reported by the Byzantine historian Justin, who, apparently relying on older sources, told us that his guardians "tried to cut him off by poison. He, however, being on his guard against treachery, frequently took antidotes, and so fortified himself by exquisite preventives against their malice." Young Mithridates, it appears, had noticed that something was amiss; perhaps there was a queer taste to his food. In his circumstances this was not an unlikely occurrence. At the Pontic court, it seems that murder by slow poison had become such a matter of routine that it always followed the same course. One particular poison was employed in small cumulative doses that were guaranteed to bring death with all the symptoms of natural disease. Some physicians believed that they had discovered an antidote to this poison. The young prince took a regular daily dose of this antidote. In fact, he continued his regimen until the day of his death. Each day, after taking his antidote, he would then take a small dose of poison to make sure that the antidote had been properly compounded. Once this routine was established, he found that he could eat, without any ill effects, the most elaborate recipes of the palace cooks.

Even after he assumed the throne his interest in poisons continued. He knew that there was more than one poison, and to be safe he would need more than just one antidote. Of the ancient medical authors, Galen, later to be so strongly denounced by Paracelsus, had the greatest interest in pharmacology and poison antidotes. In the opening part of his *De Antidotis*, Galen stated that Mithridates was zealous to have empirical or experimental knowledge of almost all the simple drugs that could be used to combat poisons. In order to obtain this information, he tested poisons and antidotes on condemned criminals. Through such experimentation Mithridates found drugs that were effective against various poisons of spiders, scorpions, and vipers. Other agents appeared to counteract other poisons also known to be lethal, such as those of aconite and of sea slugs. By mixing all of these together, Mithridates created a single medication that he hoped would provide protection against all poisons. Subsequently, Andromachus, by adding several ingredients and removing others, prepared the antidote called theriac. This featured a considerable amount of the flesh of vipers, a component that was absent from the original mithridate. Galen, without any experimental data, on only a theoretical basis, believed that theriac was better for viper bites than was the mithridate. Later, Galen gave actual recipes for making the mithridate and another antidote known as a panacea. Two other ancient writers with great interest in medicine also discussed Mithridates and his mithridate: Celsus and Pliny. The former, whose name may have been the basis of the name Paracelsus, listed the 36 ingredients of the mithridate, by which "by daily ingestion the king is said to have his body safe against the dangers of poisons." Pliny, on the other hand, complained that the mithridatic antidote was composed of 54 ingredients, no two of which had the same weight. "Which of the gods, in the name of Truth, fixed these absurd proportions," he asked, and he concluded that "it is plainly a showy parade of the art, and a colossal boast of science."

How successful was the original mithridate? Perhaps the story of the death of Mithridates is the best evidence regarding the efficacy of his regimen. With no hope left for him, Mithridates decided to kill himself with Pontic poison that he had hidden in the pommel of his sword. First he gave small doses to his two daughters, who wanted to die with him. The poison took effect on them at once, and they died quickly and painlessly. They had never needed to take the antidote during their protected, sheltered lives. The old king swallowed what was left in his sword hilt. He walked rapidly about the room to encourage the poison to flow through his veins. But more than 50 years of the daily antidote had immunized his body, and the drug failed to affect him. At last he understood he could not die by poison. There was still in his following a Gallic nobleman named Bituitus. This Bituitus was a chieftain of Galatia who had stood by his lord to the last. Mithridates turned to him, reminding him that for many years he had relied on his sharp sword and strong right arm. "But although I have been on my guard against all the poisons that a man may take with his food, I have neglected to provide against that most deadly, to be found in every royal palace: the treason of soldiers, of sons, and of friends." All other alternatives having failed, Mithridates ordered Bituitus to kill him. Obeying orders to the last, Bituitus cut him down.

Afraid that his enemies wanted to poison him, Paracelsus did just what Mithridates had done 1,500 years earlier. He protected himself by taking a mithridate. Perhaps his reliance on ancient authorities and knowledge was not as slight as he claimed.

The use of mithridates continued long after Paracelsus, not dying out until the eighteenth century. It was perhaps the great English physician William Heberden who pulled the final curtain on this drama in his essay "Antitheriaka, an Essay on Mithridatium and Theriaca," published in 1745, more than 1,800 years after the death of Mithridates VI Eupator. Heberden, like Pliny, was bothered by the great number of ingredients and even more by their often contradictory effects. He was also skeptical of the relationship between Mithridates and the mithridate as he knew it: "There is some reason to suspect that Mithridates was as much a stranger to his own antidote, as several eminent physicians have since been to the medicines that are daily advertised under their names."

When he died in Salzburg, Paracelsus was buried in the church of St. Sebastian, and his grave was marked by a simple epitaph: "Here lies Philippus Paracelsus, the famous Doctor Medicinae, who, by his wonderful art, cured bad wounds, lepra, gout, dropsy and other incurable diseases, and to his honor divided his possessions among the poor."

It is ironic but perhaps fitting that William Shakespeare forever linked the names of Paracelsus and Galen. In Scene 3, Act II, of All's Well That Ends Well, Parolles speaks of physicians: "So I say." He is seconded by Lafew: "Both of Galen and

Paracelsus." In Shakespeare's day, Galen and Paracelsus were more than just two dead physicians. They were the founders of two antagonistic schools of medicine, one that relied on ancient authorities and one that relied on empiricism. The founders themselves were more often in agreement than were their followers, and nowhere were they more united than in their view of the value of mithridates.

NOTES

Biographical sketches of Paracelsus appear in virtually every history of medicine. The splendid book by B. L. Gordon, *Medieval and Renaissance Medicine* (New York: Philosophical Library, 1959), puts his career into historical perspective.

Information on Mithridates VI is not as readily available. The best summary of his life can be found in Volume 9 of the *Cambridge Ancient History*. The best ancient source is Appian, who lived in the second century and wrote a Roman history that is primarily a history of the wars of Rome, including the important Mithridatic wars. Plutarch's accounts of the lives of Sulla, Lucullus, and Pompeius all mention Mithridates. Alfred Duggan's historical biography, *He Died Old, Mithridates Eupator, King of Pontus* (London: Peter Davies, 1958) tells his whole story in brilliant fashion. Saul Jarcho (*Bulletin of the New York Academy of Medicine* 48:1059–1063, 1972) summarized much of what is recorded by ancient historians and physicians about the pharmaceutical interests of Mithridates VI.

A Nobel Prize for Psychiatry

Oh, give me the free'n'easy
Waltz that is Viennesey–
And, go tell the band
If they want a hand
The waltz must be Strauss's.

Ira Gershwin, "By Strauss," from *The
Show Is On* (1936)

A Nobel Prize for Psychiatry

In retrospect it seems quite natural that the first Nobel prize in medicine to be given to a psychiatrist was awarded to a Viennese psychiatrist. The time was right. The place was right. The accomplishment was right. The year was 1927, and the award was part of the growing worldwide recognition of the significance of work carried out in the first two decades of this century. The place was Vienna. Vienna, which had long been famous for numerous advances in psychiatry, was becoming even more renowned as the birthplace and home of psychoanalysis. The names of Gall, Mesmer, von Feuchtersleben, Meynert, and Krafft-Ebing, who had made Vienna the stronghold of psychiatry in the nineteenth century, were being replaced by the names of Freud and his disciples. The Nobel prize was given in recognition of a great advance in psychotherapy, undoubtedly the first such great advance.

Despite its shifting political fortunes, Vienna in the 1920s was still one of the world's cultural centers. As the capital of Austria, Vienna during the first decades of the twentieth century was still basking in the glory of its years as the center of the Hapsburg Empire. In the years before the Great War, Vienna had been in many ways the cultural mecca of Europe. It was a city of great intellectual and artistic ferment. In spite of its unhurried pace and proverbial carelessness, the culture of Vienna was anything but lazy. Profundity of thought and persistence in the pursuit of ideas, both old and new, were cherished and rewarded. The long reign of Franz Joseph (1848–1916) represented the quintessence of Austrian culture, a high point in the expression of Austrian genius enriched by a cross-fertilization of peoples from throughout the Austro-Hungarian Empire and flavored by a vague awareness that all too soon this way of life would be no more. Vienna was the city of Schönberg and his students Berg and Webern, who were reshaping the structure of harmony. At the same time, it was the city of Mahler and Richard Strauss, those last great voices of postromanticism. It was still the city of the waltz, perhaps best reflected in the Strauss-Hofmannsthal masterpiece *Der Rosenkavalier*. In this opera, all the beauty, all the opulence, all the banality, all the baroque trimming, all the psychological insight of Vienna came together for a brief moment that now has a life of its own. The Marshalin understands the message of the times. She still presides over her court and courtiers, but she knows that life and history have moved beyond her. The Marshalin's bittersweet farewell to Octavian in the last scene may be more a nostalgic parting with the way of life that was Vienna than a last *auf Wiedersehen* to a young lover. In the theater, Max Reinhardt was revolutionizing stage production, as Mahler was opera production. Modern functional architecture and interior design were being shaped by Hoffman, Wagner, and Loos. In literature, Hauptmann, Stefan Zweig, Hofmannsthal, and Schnitzler were exerting an influence felt throughout the world. It must have been impossible for contemporaries to realize that this brilliant flowering was the last desperate gasp of a dying world, a world of yesterday as out of date in the 1920s as the Austro-Hungarian cavalry had been during the Great War.

Vienna meant more than the humanities. The city was unrivaled as a medical center, a postgraduate medical school for much of the world. The so-called New Vienna School founded by Rokitansky and Skoda had lost none of its magnetism.

The medical school of the University of Vienna, like the university itself, dates back to 1365. In that year, Duke Rudolph IV of Austria obtained permission from Pope Clement IV to establish a university in Vienna. This was done by converting the ancient school of St. Stephen into a university according to the ordinances and customs observed first at Athens, then at Rome, and later at Paris. During the first 400 years of its existence it was not much of a medical school. During the early years, teaching consisted entirely of reading ancient treatises to the students, predominantly those of Galen, Rhazes, and Avicenna. After 2 years of studying these masters, the successful student received a B.A. degree in medicine, unencumbered by such problems as anatomic dissections or actual contact with patients. Patient contact began in the third year and consisted of a 2- to 3-year apprenticeship with one of the physicians of the Vienna region. This apprenticeship and the writing of a dissertation on one of the aphorisms of Hippocrates had to be completed in order for the student to receive his doctorate. Surgery, of course, was beneath the dignity of such physicians.

Despite the changes that swept across European medical education in the early sixteenth century as part of the Renaissance, the medical faculty of Vienna remained a stagnant backwater. Foreign students no longer traveled to Vienna. The sons of wealthy Austrians went abroad to study. In 1629, the university was placed under the authority of the College of Jesuits, and in 1703 an imperial edict suspended the granting of medical degrees because of the poor level of medical education.

Things began to improve when Empress Maria Theresa put Gerard von Swietan (1700–1772) in charge of medical education in Austria. Swietan was a disciple of Hermann Boerhoave, and he stressed careful patient observation and common sense. Under Swietan, the medical school became a true seat of medical education to which both Austrian and foreign students flocked. In the first half of the nineteenth century the accomplishments of Corvisart, Laennec, and their students put Paris in the forefront of medicine and medical education, and by 1840, Vienna, following the Parisian methods, became the first great German-speaking medical center. Carl August Wunderlich, a youthful member of the medical faculty from Tübingen who had visited both Paris and Vienna, wrote:

> I believe I am entitled to regard as a new school this fresh trend of research in German medicine which, though originated by one man, has found zealous helpers, and which is impressive, not perhaps because of the number of its representatives, but because of their quality and the momentous character of their production. And I believe that I do wrong to no one when I style by the name of the young Viennese school the peculiarities of these able investigators, who, though each of them works in his own original way, display a quality which is unmistakably common to them all.

The one man most responsible for this new school was Carl Rokitansky (1804–1878). Rokitansky was a Czech born in Königgratz. He studied medicine first at

Prague and then at Vienna, where he received his degree in 1828. After graduation Rokitansky immediately went to work in the pathology laboratory, where he remained throughout his entire career. He became director of the Pathological Institute in 1832 and full professor in 1844. His first autopsy, on a cirrhotic composer named Beethoven, was performed in 1827. When he retired 48 years later he and his assistants had performed 59,786 such postmortem examinations. His accomplishments were many. He was the first to differentiate lobar and lobular pneumonia:

> Inflammation of the Lungs (Pneumoniae). Pathologists are in the habit of recognising only one form of pneumonia. It is true that this is by far the most frequent form: but even in regard to this there are several points which we cannot agree with the accepted view. We may provisionally and very briefly remark that the evidence of its croupous nature will be the more manifest in proportion to the epidemic constitution and the special cause of the disease, the rapidity of its course, the degree of its intensity, etc. We shall treat of this, the most common form of pneumonia, under the designation of:
>
> 1. *Croupous Pneumonia.*—The course of this disease is divided, as is well known, into three stages which have received the names of inflammatory engorgement, hepatisation, and purulent infiltration. We shall first consider the case in which a whole lung, or at least a whole lobe, is affected.
>
> Pneumonia, according to its variety, attacks, as we have already described, the whole of one of the larger divisions of the lung, that is to say, a whole lobe, or a great part of one, and it is then termed lobar.
>
> Or it attacks only smaller portions of the lungs, a number of individualized lobules or single aggregations of lobules, between which we find the parenchyma in a comparatively normal state. It is then termed lobular pneumonia.

This description appeared in his landmark textbook *A Manual of Pathological Anatomy*, published originally in German in 1842 as *Handbuch der pathologischen Anatomie*. It was translated into English by the Sydenham Society and published in four volumes that appeared between 1849 and 1854. This work contained his classic description of acute yellow atrophy of the liver:

> This affection is characterised by the saturated yellow colour, owing to a diffusion of bile throughout the tissue by extreme flabbiness and pulpiness, loss of granular texture, extreme rapidity in the reduction of size, which chiefly affects the vertical diameter, and consequently induces a flattening of the liver. It occurs chiefly in the early years of life, during puberty, and in the prime; it is remarkable for the rapid course it runs, for extreme tenderness of the liver, nervous attacks, and jaundice; it terminates fatally with febrile symptoms of a disorganized state of the blood, irritation of the brain.

It also contained his discussion of the development of emphysema:

> It presents many varieties in degree and extent. By degree, we refer to the extent of the dilatation of the pulmonary cells; it must however, be remarked, that in emphysema of long standing, we always simultaneously find several degrees of dilatation, and that it is only during the commencement of the disease that the dilatation is observed to be uniform. The pulmonary cells may be dilated to the size of a milletseed or pin's head, or to that of a hemp-seed, or pea, or even a bean, and in proportion to the size which they attain, they deviate the more from their original shape. At first the disease is a genuine, simple dilatation of the cells,

and when the cell walls become to a certain extent thickened and rigid, it may be regarded as an active dilatation of the cells somewhat analogous to hypertrophy of the lungs. In higher degrees, on the contrary, the dilated cells unite to form a larger space, their walls becoming atrophied by the pressure they exert on one another.

This and other major works, such as *Defects of the Valves of the Heart*, published in 1875, and *Diseases of the Arteries*, published in 1852, modernized the entire field of pathology. His 1842 *Handbuch* was the most influential of these. This medical classic not only contained a wealth of material with excellent descriptions and illustrations of both gross and microscopic pathologic changes but perhaps even more significantly contained a clear and logical classification of diseases based on pathology. It was because of this that Virchow referred to Rokitansky as the "Linne of pathologic anatomy."

In 1849 Rokitansky was appointed dean of the medical faculty, and the following year he became rector of the university. He was an outstanding teacher, and he attracted students from near and far to the pathology amphitheater. In this setting he brought about a quiet revolution in medical education. For centuries patients had been treated and had died, and no systematic attempt had been made to perform autopsies and correlate the pathologic findings with patients' medical histories. In Vienna, autopsies became part of the legally prescribed routine, and under Rokitansky both clinicians and pathologists participated in autopsies. His success in bringing practicing physicians into the study of postmortem findings set a precedent we still follow.

Once they were at the autopsy table, clinicians could for the first time learn of their triumphs and failures. More significantly, after such study Rokitansky could classify anatomic lesions and relate them to clinically recorded signs and symptoms. Anatomic pathology, as propounded by Rokitansky, revealed the natural history of the morbid process, the progress of the clinical course of disease consonant with the structural changes.

Joseph Skoda (1805–1881), a fellow Bohemian, was the best-known clinician of the New Viennese School. Self-taught in the recently developed techniques of auscultation and percussion, he carefully percussed and auscultated patients and then went to watch Rokitansky's postmortem examinations. In 1839 he published his monograph "Abhandlung über Perkussion und Auskultation," which in many respects constituted the cornerstone of modern physical diagnosis.

The school founded by Rokitansky and Skoda and carried forward by their associates and students soon usurped the preeminence of Paris. By the middle decades of the nineteenth century there was a widespread belief that no European doctor's education was complete unless he had spent a considerable period studying in Vienna. Not only Europeans felt the attraction; Americans began to include Vienna in their tours of Old World postgraduate training centers. Olser studied in Vienna, as did many others. As the nineteenth century gave way to the twentieth, American physicians continued to flock to Vienna. At one time it was almost as if no self-respecting American specialist was considered worthy of the title specialist unless he had studied in Vienna.

It was in this milieu that a Viennese psychiatrist revolutionized the treatment of the most widespread and most dreaded of all psychiatric diseases and received a well-deserved Nobel prize for medicine. His name became a household word. His face even appeared on an Austrian banknote. His name? Not Sigmund Freud, but Wagner von Jauregg. His contribution: fever therapy for general paresis of the insane. General paresis of the insane (GPI or parenchymatous neurosyphilis) is a progressive, uniformly fatal mental illness developed by some patients 5 to 20 years after their original syphilitic infections. General paretics are rare in mental hospitals today, but at one time they constituted a large proportion of mental hospital populations, one of the reasons that Kraepelin, in his classic study of schizophrenia, took GPI as his model form of insanity.

Syphilis is generally believed to have become common in Europe in the sixteenth century, but general paresis was not recognized as a clinical entity until the 1820s. Syphilis as an acute infection seems to have first appeared in Europe shortly after the return of Christopher Columbus and his crew. Whether the dissemination was due to the activities of the former or the latter remains open to conjecture.

The New World origin of syphilis, which was accepted by almost all contemporary authorities, has recently come under attack. The history of the spread of the disease and the observations of late fifteenth- and sixteenth-century physicians and historians make a strong case for the so-called Haitian hypothesis. This hypothesis states that Columbus's crew consorted with native women in Haiti, contracted the disease, and brought it back with them to Spain, from where it spread throughout Europe.

A military campaign played a major role in spreading this devastating new disease. In the fall of 1494, Charles VIII, king of France, invaded Italy in an attempt to enforce his claim to the throne of the Kingdom of Naples. Italy was then divided into numerous city-states and petty kingdoms that had been weakened by constant internecine rivalry. Thus Charles met no effective resistance during his initial advance into Italy, and his army easily marched down the peninsula to Naples. His army was composed of mercenaries from all parts of western Europe, including French, German, Swiss, English, Hungarian, Polish, Italian, and, of course, Spanish troops. This 30,000-man force was accompanied by some 900 camp followers. In most instances the camp followers were prostitutes. The march to Naples was more a parade of debauchery than a serious military campaign. In late 1494 Charles and his army began their siege of Naples. What happened next is easy to imagine. In army camps at that time, sexual diversion was an expected and welcome change of pace. The women often moved freely from one side to the other, and Spanish mercenaries were serving in Charles's army as well as among the defenders of Naples. Given these circumstances, the spread of the new venereal disease is easy to comprehend. Fallopius, the great anatomist who lived from 1523 to 1562 and whose father lived in Naples during the siege, told how the defenders of Naples "finally with violence drove their harlots and women out of the citadel, and especially the most beautiful ones, whom they knew to be suffering from the infectious disease, on the pretext that the food had come to an end. And the French, gripped by compassion and bewitched by their beauty, took them in." By the spring of 1495 this new disease accomplished something the Neapolitans could not: Charles's army was devastated, and he was forced to abandon his campaign and retreat. The withdrawal back up the Italian peninsula presented a great contrast to the almost triumphant advances of the previous fall. Charles's army disintegrated into undisciplined lawless bands that fled northward and scattered into France, Switzerland, Germany, and their other homelands, bringing their new disease with them. In recognition of the source of the disaster, the new affliction was first called Neapolitan disease, but it soon became known as the French disease. Charles VIII himself died from it in 1498 at the age of only 28.

Virtually all contemporary records mention the explosive spread of the disease, which later became known as syphilis. They all agree in attributing the epidemic to Charles's army and its dissemination to the scattering of his troops. The spread of syphilis from Italy can be traced in the local chronicles of the time, step by step with the dispersal of Charles's army. It appeared in France, Germany, and Switzerland in 1495, in Holland and Greece in 1496. It spread to England and Scotland in 1497, to Hungary and Russia in 1499.

The first spread of the disease to the Orient is not as well documented, but the available records suggest that Vasco da Gama's men took it to Calcutta, India, from where it spread to the Malay peninsula, which even then was an important trading center. From Malay it spread, at the beginning of the sixteenth century, to Canton, and in China it became known as Canton disease. When syphilis reached Kyoto, Japan, it was given the name *karakasa*, Chinese pleasure disease.

Some medical historians are of the opinion that syphilis was present in Europe and elsewhere from the days of antiquity. According to these authors, the French march on Naples involving camp followers and abundant opportunities for licentiousness merely stirred up and spread the organism and brought on its most virulent manifestations. Such a theory does not explain why this one campaign, which certainly was no more licentious than any other, resulted in this new form of a supposedly old disease.

However, there is no doubt that syphilis was at once recognized as a totally new disease. It was described as a disease usually of venereal origin that, in contrast to all other genital diseases, regularly had generalized cutaneous and systemic manifestations. The ancients had been aware of purely local genital diseases. It is striking that in all medieval and ancient sources there was not one definite reference to a venereal/genital disease with which systemic signs and symptoms were commonly seen. This peculiar feature of syphilis was recognized by contemporaries as definite evidence that this was a new disease. As Pussey pointed out in his classic *History of Syphilis*, there was no satisfactory description of the syndrome of syphilis written prior to 1493.

The severity of syphilis during its initial epidemic phase is also taken today as evidence of its newness. It is virtually an axiom in the history of diseases that when an infectious disease first appears among a people, first gains a foothold in virgin soil, it manifests itself with greater severity in terms of both morbidity and mortality than is seen among people already exposed and adapted to the disease. This has been recorded many times in many places for many diseases, including measles, scarlet fever, and smallpox, as well as in modern epidemics of syphilis among isolated peoples.

This severity was characteristic of the great epidemic of syphilis at the end of the fifteenth century. In contrast with the almost trivial character of the early manifestations of syphilis as usually seen in endemic settings, all evidence points to a severe character during this first epidemic. Most sufferers presented with an acute febrile disorder with high fever, intense headache, bone and joint pains, early skin symptoms so severe that they simulated smallpox, great prostration, and very frequently a fatal ending early in the course of the disease. Today, such a profound initial phase is rare, if not totally unknown, in nonvirginal populations. Thus, this epidemic had all the characteristics of a virulent plague. Given the morals of the time, syphilization of much of the world occurred rapidly, and many contemporaries found that the severity of the early symptoms of syphilis rapidly diminished. Within 50 years the disease assumed the character that it has today.

Several early Spanish sources documented the Haitian hypothesis. Two of these are the most important historians of the early development of the Spanish Empire: Bartolomé de las Casas (1474–1566) and Gonzalo Fernandez Oviedo (1478–1557). These two historians rarely saw things in the same light, but they agreed on one thing: syphilis was of New World origin. Las Casas was in Seville in 1493 when Columbus arrived from the New World. His father and uncle accompanied Columbus on his second voyage later that year. Later Las Casas himself went to the New World and spent many years in Haiti. In his famous *Historia de las Indias* he described syphilis, known in Italy as the French malady, as one of the great dangers that the New World held for Spaniards:

> This, let it be known in truth, was taken from this island, either when the first Indians left at the time of Admiral D. Christobal Colon returned with the news of the discovery of the Indies, which men I saw myself soon afterwards in Seville, and these were in a position to communicate it to Spain, by infecting the air or in other ways [what a pointed warning]; or when some Spaniards having already contracted the disease went on the first return voyage to Castile, and this could have happened between the years 1494 to 96; and because at this time King Charles of France, whom they call the Bighead, passed with a great army into Italy, to take Naples, and that contagious malady was in that army—for this reason the Italians thought that they had caught it from them, and from then on they called it the French disease. I myself sometimes endeavored to inquire of the Indians of this island if this malady were very ancient in it, and they answered yes. . . . It is a thing well verified that all the incontinent Spaniards that did not have the virtue of chastity on this island were contaminated by it (recall, gentlemen, the clear warning that I brought to your attention a few moments ago), and out of a hundred perhaps not one escaped except when the other party never had it.
>
> The Indians, men or women, that had it were little affected by it, almost as little as if they only had smallpox.

Oviedo was attached to the Spanish court and had met Columbus prior to his voyage to the New World. He was in Barcelona when Columbus returned there in

1493. He asked a number of his friends who sailed on subsequent voyages with Columbus to bring back detailed reports to him. In 1513 he traveled to the Indies and spent much of the rest of his life there. In his *Historia General y Natural de las Indias*, which was published in 1535, he proclaimed that syphilis was contracted by the Spanish sailors from Indian women and brought back to Spain, from where it was distributed to the army of Charles VIII by Spanish mercenaries, presumably via third parties: "Many times in Italy I laughed, hearing the Italians speak of the French disease, and the French call it the disease of Naples; and in truth both would have had the name better if they called it the disease of the Indies."

A third Spanish source for the Haitian hypothesis was a physician named Ruiz Diaz de Isla (1462–1542), whose *Tractado centra el mal serpentino* was written between 1510 and 1520 and published in 1539. Diaz was a well-known physician at the Hospital of All Saints in Lisbon. In this position he treated some of Columbus's original crew, as well as others who contracted the disease as it spread through the Iberian peninsula. Originally he did not know what the disease was, but he later realized that he had witnessed the arrival of a new disease, which he called *morbo serpentino*. The lengthy title of his book was originally translated as "Treatise on the serpentine malady, which in Spain is commonly called bubas, which was drawn up in the hospital of All Saints in Lisbon . . . printed in the very noble and very loyal city of Seville, in the house of Domenico de Robertis, printer of books. Finished the twenty-seventh of September, MDXXXIX."

In his treatise he stated that the new disease (only later called syphilis) was unknown before 1493 and was brought to Spain by the crew of Columbus on their return from the first voyage to Española (Haiti). Diaz called it the disease of the isle of Española, but he also gave a number of native names for the disease. A majority of Columbus's crew returned to Spain infected with syphilis, and Diaz himself treated several syphilitic sailors, including Pincon of Palos.

> It has pleased divine justice to give and send down upon us unknown afflictions, never seen nor recognized nor found in medical books, such as the serpentine disease. . . . At the time that the admiral don Xristobal Colon arrived in Spain the Catholic sovereigns were in the city of Barcelona. And when they went to give them an account of their voyage and of what they had discovered, immediately the city began to be infected and the aforesaid disease spread, as was seen later on through long experience.

Perhaps the most interesting attribution of the French disease to the New World was that of Nicholas Monardes. Monardes, in his *Joyfull Newes Out of the New Founde Worlde*, logically demonstrated that syphilis had to have originated in the New World. Monardes firmly believed that God in his infinite mercy always placed a remedy for a disease near its source. He also believed that guaiacum, made from a West Indian wood, was a sure cure for the French disease. Thus if guaiacum cured syphilis, syphilis must have originated in the West Indies: "Our Lorde GOD would from whence this euill of the Poxe came, from thence would come the remedy for them." Unfortunately, guaiacum, known as the "holy wood," had little if any efficacy.

How, then, did syphilis, the French disease, the Neapolitan disease, the morbo serpentino, get its name? It received its name about 1530 in a poem by Girolamo Fracastoro (1478–1553) entitled "Syphilis sive morbus gallicus." Fracastoro was a true son of the Italian Renaissance. Although medicine was his greatest interest, he also studied astronomy, physics, mathematics, geology, geography, and botany, and, of course, he was a poet of some note. He was born in Verona but went to the University of Padua, the leading medical school of the day, where his fellow students included several future cardinals and a young Pole named Niklas Koppernigk, who posthumously became better known as an astronomer than as a physician. After finishing his studies he returned to his villa near Verona, where he spent most of his life studying and writing. He did practice medicine, at first only treating members of the local peasantry, but later, as his reputation as a scholar, humanist, and physician grew, he was sought out by patients from near and far. His famous poem probably was written in one of his lighter moments, and it added myth to the knowledge that had been gathered concerning the new disease. The myth was that a shepherd named Syphilus was struck with the disease because he had blasphemed the Sun God. The name Syphilus, like the myth, may have been the product of Fracastoro's imagination, or he may have derived it from the Greek word for shameful or repulsive. There is even some evidence that the word *syphilis* had been used colloquially around Verona and that the name *Syphilus* came from this slang term *syphilis*. In any case, the poem, which was one of the most obscene poems to appear in any literature, was a success. It spread as rapidly as the French disease, and in the end it resulted in a new name for the new pestilence. The knowledge the poet compiled was as significant as the obscene passages he included in his poem:

> In some persons, the disease commenced without contagion; in others, and these were the greater number, it was transmitted by contagion. Not every kind of contact sufficed for producing it; it required that two bodies should become heated together, as occurs in the act of coition. And it was chiefly by coition that the greatest number became infected. However, a considerable number of children contracted the disease by sucking their diseased mothers or nurses. The disease was not communicable at a distance; it did not show itself immediately, but sometimes at the end of one, two, or even four months; certain signs, however, announced already that the disease was in germ.
>
> Those affected were sad, weary and cast-down; they were pale; most of them had sores on the genital organs, ulcers similar to those which are wont to develop themselves on these organs after coition, and which are called caries, but of a very different nature; they were obstinate. When they were cured in one place, they appeared in another, and the treatment had to be recommenced. Afterwards, pustules arose on the skin, covered with a crust; in some they appeared upon the head, which was the most frequent place; in others they appeared elsewhere. At first they were small; afterwards they increased to the size of an acorn, which they resembled in shape, their appearance otherwise being similar to the crusta lactea of children. In some cases these pustules were small and dry. In others they were large and moist; in some livid; in others whitish and rather pale; in others hard and reddish. They always broke in a few days, and constantly discharged an incredible quantity of stinking matter as soon as open; they were so many true

phagedaenic ulcers, which destroyed not only the flesh, but even the bones. Those attacked in the upper parts of the body suffered from malignant affection, which eat away sometimes the palate, sometimes the fauces, sometimes the larynx, sometimes the tonsils; some lost the lips, others the nose, others all the genital organs. Many had gummy tumors on the limbs, which disfigured them, and were often the size of an egg, or of a small loaf; when they broke, a kind of white mucilaginous fluid flowed from them. They attacked chiefly the arms and legs; sometimes they remained callous until death.

But, as if all this were not sufficient, there ensued, moreover, severe pains in the limbs, often at the same time with the pustules; sometimes before, sometimes after them. These pains, which were persistent and unbearable, were chiefly felt in the night, and were seated in the limbs themselves, and in the nerves rather than in the joints; some, however, had pustules without the pains, others pains without the pustules; most had both pustules and pains. However, all the limbs were in a languid condition; the patients were wan and emaciated, without appetite, sleepless, always melancholy and ill-humored, and anxious to remain in bed. Their faces and legs swelled, and a slow fever sometimes supervened, but rarely. Some suffered pains in the head, which were persistent, and did not yield to any remedy. If blood was drawn, it was found to be pure, and somewhat mucous; the urine was thick and red; by this sign alone, supervening in the absence of fever, the disease might be recognized; the stools were liquid and mucous.

Such were the symptoms of the disease at its commencement; but I speak of a past time, for now, although the disease is still prevalent, it nevertheless appears to differ from what it was then. We have seen during about the last twenty years, fewer pustules and more gummy tumors, which is the reverse of what was observed in the first years. The pustules, when any appear, are drier, and the pains, when supervene, more severe. Within six years the disease has again changed notably; we now see pustules in but very few patients; scarcely any pains, or much slighter ones, but many gummy tumors.

This poem was not Fracastoro's only significant contribution to medicine. His interest in syphilis led him to study other contagious diseases, and his years of study culminated in the publication of another book, *De Contagione*, in 1546. Fracastoro, in this book, defined contagion as "an infection that passes from one thing to another." He distinguished three types of contagion: "contagion that infects by contact only," "contagion that infects by fomites," and "contagion at a distance." He recognized the contagiousness of such diseases as smallpox, measles, tuberculosis, rabies, and, of course, syphilis, and he was the first to recognize typhus. He died in 1553 of a massive stroke and was buried in Verona. There a statue was erected in honor of the author of the divine poem about Syphilus (Fig. 1).

Syphilis as a widespread disease in western Europe dates back to the 1490s, but GPI was not known until some 300 years later. If syphilis had settled down to an endemic form by the time of Fracastoro, how can we explain this late recognition of neurosyphilis? The delay of 300 years between the recognition of acute syphilis and that of GPI cannot be due solely to the long latency period of the disease. The final recognition of GPI as a specific disease may have occurred in the early years of the nineteenth century as a result of many factors. First, there was, by then, increased interest in insanity. This was associated historically with the teachings of Esquirol (1772–1840), who emphasized the value of observation and detailed

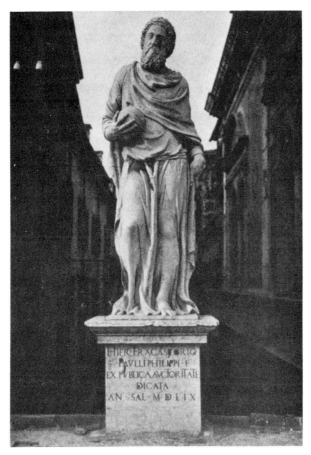

FIG. 1.   Statue of Girolamo Fracastoro by Danese Cattaneo, erected on the Piazza dei Signori in Verona, Italy, in 1559. (From Ralph H. Major, *A History of Medicine*, 1954. Courtesy of Charles C Thomas, Springfield, Ill.)

case recording and stressed the need to break down the old trinity of madness (mania, melancholia, dementia) into discrete homogeneous illnesses. The establishment of mental hospitals made it possible for patients with adverse prognoses to be observed over long periods of time. Finally, the study of pathologic anatomy stimulated postmortem examinations of the brain. General paresis, a common mental illness with such distinct features as epilepsy, paralysis, and dementia, which were based on specific pathological lesions, at last brought psychiatry to the same level as other branches of medicine in which signs and symptoms were being associated with specific structural abnormalities. Syphilis even became the model psychiatric disease, with attempts being made to find analogous conditions and establish other entities like Kraepelin's concept of dementia praecox fashioned along the lines of "dementia paralytica." All of these factors might explain why syphilis of the central nervous system was not recognized for 300 years. But perhaps not. It is also possible that GPI was not recognized during this period because it did not exist as a disease entity.

The failure to recognize GPI between the arrival of syphilis at the end of the fifteenth century and the first clinical reports of the disease in the 1820s could have been due to its virtual absence during this period. How could such an absence of a natural phase of syphilis be explained? Perhaps nature had anticipated von Jauregg and used the same method he did, the induction of recurrent high fevers to prevent the occurrence of GPI.

A large number of infectious diseases associated with high fevers were endemic in Europe during the fifteenth, sixteenth, seventeenth, eighteenth, and even nineteenth centuries. These included malaria, smallpox, relapsing fever, typhus, and others. These could all have played roles. Diaz de Isla, in 1539, suggested that a high fever such as that caused by malaria tended to arrest syphilis. At one time, malaria was a common disease in Europe. Pandemics of malaria recurred for centuries after the introduction of syphilis, the last appearing between 1855 and 1873.

It is reasonable to assume that better methods of treatment (first cinchona bark and then quinine) shortened the duration of malaria in many cases in the later pandemics and reduced the prophylactic effect of malaria-induced fever by the nineteenth century. The prophylactic efficacy of epidemic and endemic malaria can best be appreciated by looking outside of Europe, where there is fairly convincing evidence that widespread malaria in various areas provides the populations of those regions with reasonable protection against the late neurologic complications of syphilis.

But malaria is not the only prophylactic fever and probably has not been the most important means of prevention. Smallpox probably also played a major role. As we shall see later, it helped to stimulate von Jauregg's imagination.

Smallpox is characterized by two distinct bouts of fever. The first involves temperatures up to 41°C or 42°C for 3 or 4 days during the prodromal stage. Then, if the case is uncomplicated, a second episode of milder fever for 9 or 10 days occurs during the stages of eruption. Because of these characteristics, smallpox should provide excellent protection against general paresis. Thus the question must be raised whether or not smallpox was sufficiently common in Europe prior to the end of the eighteenth century and the widespread introduction of vaccination to have afforded protection from GPI. It certainly was. Smallpox was reported to have killed 45 million of Europe's 165 million inhabitants in the eighteenth century. One of every 400 Europeans died each year of smallpox, and at least 1 of 3 Europeans got the disease. Statisticians today would add the term *competitive mortality* in any description of this form of protection. With the birth of modern medicine and large-scale vaccination against smallpox, the smallpox rate declined, and as it did, more and more general paresis began to appear. The negative correlation between these two diseases has been observed both inside and outside Europe, and it is striking, to say the least.

This was best documented in 1926, the year before Wagner von Jauregg won his Nobel prize, by a Ukrainian psychiatrist named Daraszkiewicz. He was a well-trained psychiatrist who had worked for several years under Kraepelin, and he reported that during 15 years of practice in the Ukraine he had not seen a single paretic with scars after smallpox. During this same time he saw such scars in many patients suffering from other mental diseases. Moreover, he had never seen a paretic without a scar from vaccination. His conclusion, based on these observations, was twofold. First, he believed that unvaccinated persons could hardly avoid contracting smallpox and that this gave them "absolute" protection against GPI. Second, he believed that syphilis could not lead to general paresis unless the victim had been "tainted" with cowpox, that is, vaccinated against smallpox.

Daraszkiewicz drew attention to the observation that there was practically no general paresis in Europe from 1500 to 1800, although syphilis was common, and that the same was still true in areas not yet touched by European civilization and its associated vaccinations. Daraszkiewicz was widely attacked for his views, and although his contention that vaccination made syphilis more neurotrophic remains unproven, the protective role of smallpox seems clear.

Relapsing fevers, a group of infectious diseases, have been used therapeutically to treat GPI with some efficacy, but because they are themselves difficult to control, they have never been widely used as therapy for GPI. However, such naturally occurring infections would be expected to have a prophylactic value. In Europe, relapsing fever is usually transmitted by lice, whereas outside of Europe it is spread by ticks. Epidemics occurred in various parts of Europe in the eighteenth century and in Russia and Ireland in the nineteenth century, and during recent decades large epidemics have occurred in central and southern Europe and in North Africa. Many non-European countries continue to suffer from endemic relapsing fever. Undoubtedly, this disease also played a role, at significant cost, in preventing GPI.

Tick-borne typhus, an epidemic rickettsial disease first described by Fracastoro, most likely played an even greater part in preventing GPI, at a much greater cost. Typhus is characterized by prolonged high fever, sometimes lasting for as long as 10 days. This has a strongly deleterious effect on *Treponema pallidum*. Young people seldom die of the disease, but the mortality rises with age to over 60%. The disease is spread by lice and is especially prevalent during times of war. It caused great havoc in Europe in the seventeenth and eighteenth centuries, and a widespread epidemic developed in the wake of Napoleon's retreat from Moscow in 1812 and spread over most of Europe. Other fever-causing diseases may also have been of some value in this regard, including typhoid fever and related disorders. The high-fever diseases were so common that there was little chance of anyone escaping them all and not receiving the benefit of their protective powers.

These fevers also have a less specific effect, that of competitive mortality. In the years between 1500 and 1800 it was common for otherwise healthy adults to die suddenly of acute infectious diseases, often during the incubation period of GPI. Only as these diseases disappeared did enough people live long enough to make GPI common enough to be recognized as part of a mixed blessing from increased public health measures aimed at increasing life expectancy.

Finally GPI was recognized, as were other central nervous system manifestations of syphilis, and by the late nineteenth century these were rampant. Great advances were made in the diagnosis of syphilis, but treatment lagged far behind the diagnostic advances. Paul Ehrlich (1854–1915) introduced 606 (salvarsan, neoarsphenamine) in the treatment of syphilis in 1910. This "salvation" arsenical was found in his 606th experiment and thus was given the name 606. It was unique in that it destroyed spirochetes within the patient's body. Despite its efficacy in the early stages of syphilis, salvarsan was of little value in GPI.

Julius Wagner von Jauregg (1857–1940) must get full credit for developing the first truly effective form of therapy of central nervous system syphilis. He was born in Wels, Austria. His father was a state official there. His name was Wagner until he was knighted and added the von Jauregg. Wagner von Jauregg studied medicine at the University of Vienna, receiving his degree in 1880. After graduation he continued to work in the Institute of Pathology until 1883, when he accepted a position in a psychiatric clinic, apparently only after he failed to obtain a position in any internal medicine clinic. While working at the clinic, he discovered that several patients with mental symptoms improved after suffering acute attacks of typhoid fever. In 1887 he wrote an article suggesting the treatment of patients suffering from psychoses by infecting them with febrile disease, such as malaria or erysipelas. He attempted to treat some of these patients by injecting a culture of streptococci, but he failed to produce erysipelas. After Robert Koch discovered tuberculin, he used this to produce fever, but he abandoned it as too dangerous.

Wagner von Jauregg moved to Graz in 1889 to become head of the Department of Psychiatry of the university. Following Meynert's death in 1892, he returned to Vienna as chief of the Psychiatric Clinic of the Allgemeine Krankenhaus. In 1902 he succeeded Krafft-Ebing as professor of neurology and psychiatry at the University of Vienna. Despite increasing responsibilities and broadening interests, von Jauregg never lost sight of the possibility of treating psychosis with fever. In 1921, Mattauchek and Pilcz reported their long-term follow-up of 4,134 syphilitic officers in the Austrian Army. They noted that 4.6% eventually became paretic. They also found that not a single instance of paresis developed among the 241 officers who contracted acute infectious diseases, such as malaria, erysipelas, pneumonia, and typhoid fever, within a few years of contracting syphilis. Without any such prophylactic event, the expected number of cases of GPI among these 241 officers would have been somewhere between nine and twelve.

Wagner von Jauregg was impressed by these data and also by the observation that general paresis did not occur in countries where malaria was endemic. Finally, in 1917, he put his general theory into specific practice. In that year he inoculated "benign tertian" malaria organisms into patients with GPI. To do this, he obtained blood from the cubital veins of soldiers suffering from malaria and then injected the blood, hopefully containing malarial organisms, into other patients diagnosed as having general paresis. This procedure was not approved by any committee on human investigation, nor was any informed consent obtained, but it worked. Of the nine patients von Jauregg treated, six definitely benefited, and three of them were still at their occupations 4 years later. For his discovery of the therapeutic value of malaria inoculation in the treatment of dementia paralytica, Wagner von Jauregg was awarded the Nobel prize for physiology and medicine in 1927. He was the first psychiatrist, and to date the only psychiatrist, to receive this honor.

Von Jauregg's contributions were not limited to neurosyphilis. He wrote many papers on the relationships between mental disorders and structural diseases of the nervous system. He was also a pioneer in the prevention of cretinism, and he was the first person to suggest obligatory addition of iodide to table salt in endemic goiter areas.

Malarial therapy for GPI was soon replaced by other methods of producing high temperature. By the 1940s these all were superseded by penicillin. But none of these later advances detracts from the marvel of von Jauregg's accomplishment. When he arrived on the scene there was no rational, efficacious form of therapy for any type of psychosis. By his own observations and reasoning he virtually single-handedly gave psychiatry its first major therapeutic tool.

Von Jauregg was not the first physician to suggest the therapeutic value of induced fevers. Nor was Ruiz Diaz de Isla. This suggestion probably was first made by an earlier physician best known as a comparative anatomist, Rufus of Ephesus. Rufus was a Greek physician who lived during the reign of Trajan (98–117 C.E.). His works record the status of the subject of anatomy in Alexandria before Galen. According to his own statements, his knowledge of anatomy was derived from dissecting apes or monkeys. He complained that in his day the study of anatomy was confined to animal dissection and, at best, some examination of human surface anatomy on slaves, whereas in earlier times human bodies had been dissected for teaching purposes. His major contributions were in neuroanatomy. His book *On the Names of the Various Parts of the Body* is considered to have been the first comprehensive treatise on anatomic nomenclature. In it he presented the first description of the optic chiasma. He also traced other nerves back to the brain and differentiated between motor and sensory nerves. Anatomy was not his only interest. As a practicing physician he took great care in reaching the correct diagnosis, and in his book *On the Investigation of the Patient* he stressed especially the importance of taking an accurate history:

> It is necessary to question the patient, for by so doing one may gather more exact information concerning the nature of the malady, and will then be able to treat it more intelligently. In this way also one may learn whether the patient's mind is in a normal or an excited state, and whether any change has taken place in his physical strength. Some idea regarding the nature and seat of the disease is usually obtained from such questioning. If, for example, the patient answered clearly and to the point, and does not hesitate; if his memory does not play him false; if his speech is not thick or indistinct; if, being a well-bred man, he gives his responses in a polite cultivated manner; or if, in the case of a person who is naturally timid, the answers reflect this timidity, then you may feel confident that your patient's mind is not affected. But if, on the other hand, you ask him about one thing and he gives you a reply about something entirely different; if, as he talks, he appears to forget what he was talking about; if he has a trembling tongue the movements of which are also uncertain; and, finally, if from a certain state of

mind he passes rapidly to one of a totally different character,—all these changes are evidences that the brain is beginning to be affected. . . . If the patient speaks distinctly and with a fairly strong voice, and is able to tell his story without stopping from time to time in order to rest, the inference is warranted that his physical strength is not materially affected.

A small part of one of his 102 books (only 6 of which have come down to us intact) was preserved by Oreibasios, the friend and physician of Julian the Apostate. Oreibasios recorded that Rufus of Ephesus believed that one could not find another drug that would treat in a more penetrating manner than fever. "For this reason it is a good remedy for an individual seized with convulsion, for a patient rigid with tetanus as well as for a woman in labor with convulsions. If there were a physician skilled enough to produce a fever, it would be useless to seek any other remedy against disease."

Only 1,800 years later did von Jauregg confirm the contention of this Greek physician of the first half of the second century.

NOTES

There are so many sources on the history of syphilis that any selection of references must reflect the prejudices of the selector. Crosby's "The Early History of Syphilis" (*American Anthropologist* 71:218–227, 1969) gives a balanced appraisal of the sources. Somewhat greater documentation can be found in Mettler's *History of Medicine*, but Pussey's *The History of Epidemiology of Syphilis* (Springfield, Ill.: Thomas, 1933) remains my favorite. The only complete discussion of the inverse relationship between GPI and other infectious diseases is Bernard Jacobowsky's "General Paresis and Civilization" (*Acta Psychiatrica Scandinavica* 41:267–273, 1965). The most readily available English-language history of the Vienna School of Medicine is "Six Hundred Years of Medicine in Vienna," by Alfred Vogl, which originally appeared in the *Bulletin of the New York Academy of Medicine* (42:282–299, 1967) and was reprinted in Jarcho's *Essays and Notes on the History of Medicine* (New York: New York Academy of Medicine, 1976).

The Court-Martial of William A. Hammond

My earliest recollection of American neurology was when, as an intern in Bellevue Hospital, I became possessed of a copy of Hammond's "Treatise on Nervous Diseases" of 1874.

This was the . . . first textbook on nervous diseases in the English language. . . . To one who, like myself, was passing his days in a succession of hospital rounds percussing chests, listening to rales and cardiac bruits, testing albumin and trying to alleviate the arthritic, this work opened a new vista in the clinical and pathologic field and made a very special appeal.

Now I learned that diagnosis was not alone a matter of reaction to sense and observation, but called for reasoning and induction.

Charles L. Dana, "Early Neurology in the United States," *Journal of the American Medical Association* 90:1422–1425, 1928.

The Court-Martial of William A. Hammond

If he is remembered at all today, William Alexander Hammond (1828–1900) is recalled because of his original use of the term athetosis to define a specific class of abnormal involuntary movements. This almost automatic type of association of a name with a disorder certainly does not do full justice to this man, nor to his role in American medicine, nor, especially, to his numerous lasting contributions to American neurology. Hammond wrote the first American textbook of neurology. He was responsible for organizing the first American neurological society and was one of the founders of the American Neurological Association. He also founded what is now the Armed Forces Institute of Pathology, and with his close friend Silas Weir Mitchell he was responsible for securing a place for neurology within the American medical establishment. During a significant part of his professional life he was also known as the only surgeon general of the United States who had ever been successfully court-martialed.

In his textbook *A Treatise on Diseases of the Nervous System* (New York: D. Appleton & Co., 1871), Hammond used the Greek term *athetosis*, meaning "without fixed position," to describe a type of movement abnormality that he believed had not previously been recognized. He originally presented two cases that were characterized by "an inability to retain the fingers and toes in any position in which they might be placed and by their continual motion." He was following the first of these two patients in his own practice, and the second was a patient of Dr. J. C. Hubbard of Ashtabula, Ohio, who had sent Hammond the details of his patient's history (posthemiplegic unilateral abnormal movements), as well as photographs of the abnormal postures of the patient's hand. In both cases the movements were unilateral, predominantly involving the fingers and toes, and following an acute hemiplegia. Although he had no pathologic material to study, Hammond suggested that the lesion responsible for the abnormal movements was within the striatum:

> There is slight tremor of both upper extremities, but there is no paralysis of any part of his body. There are, however, involuntary grotesque muscular movements of the fingers and toes of the right side, and these are not those of simple flexion and extension, but of more complicated form. They occur, not only when he is awake, but also when he is asleep, and are only restrained by certain positions, and by extraordinary efforts of the will.
>
> The phenomena indicate the implication of intracranial ganglia, and the upper part of the spinal cord. The analogies of the affection are with chorea and cerebrospinal sclerosis, but it is clearly neither of these diseases. One probable seat of the morbid process is the corpus striatum.

Subsequent authors, in retrospect, have pointed out that there had been several previous reports of abnormal involuntary movements in association with hemiplegia or diplegia that most likely did represent athetosis. James Parkinson, in his classic "An Essay on the Shaking Palsy," published in London in 1817, quoted Linnaeus's description of a disorder in which there was continuous distortion of the limbs without affection of the mind that was called *morbus sacer*. Prior to Hammond's work, it had been observed that acute flaccid hemiplegia usually progressed to a spastic state and that occasionally in younger patients the acute hemiplegia was followed after a long period by spontaneous movements of the involved hand. The fingers would seem to wander from overflexion to overextension and back again. Although the terms *spasmoparalysis* and *spasmocontracture* had been applied to this syndrome, such movements generally were lumped together with chorea and were not thought of as a single pathophysiological entity.

Two years after Hammond published the report of his two patients (1873), the first description of what is now called double athetosis appeared. The claim that athetosis was a specific disorder stirred up a great deal of controversy. Not even S. Weir Mitchell, Hammond's close friend and former coinvestigator, recognized the significance of Hammond's cases. In 1874, Weir Mitchell described a patient with very similar posthemiplegic abnormal movements, and he classified the movements as "hemi chorea." Two years later, William R. Gowers, the great English clinician, reported another such patient in whom autopsy revealed a lesion of the contralateral thalamus, and he used the term *mobile spasm* to describe the movements. It should be recalled that all of these descriptions were published at a time when our understanding of the pathologic bases of movement disorders, as well as their classification, was very limited. Huntington's original description had just been published, but the pathologic basis of Huntington's chorea was still unknown (see Chapter 11). The pathology of Parkinson's disease had not yet been discovered. Other classes of abnormal movements still remained to be described. It would be some 30 years before Oppenheim would present his classic delineation of dystonia musculorum deformans (1911). Perhaps the strongest opponent of Hammond's view of athetosis as a specific phenomenon was the great Charcot, who believed that athetosis was merely a simple form of chorea. In his famous *Lectures on Diseases of the Nervous System* (1879), as translated by G. Sigerson, he attacked Hammond's original position that only the fingers and toes were involved:

> It should be added that the movements of the fingers are performed slowly, and that the fingers have a tendency to assume constraint attitudes. Moreover, the athetosis does not always remain limited to muscles which move the fingers and toes; sometimes, in fact, the entire hand and foot are affected.

Hammond did modify his initial description to include movements involving more musculature, but still characterized by relatively continuous motion. He never changed his views on the pathologic basis of athetosis, and in 1890 his son Graeme Hammond presented the finding on necropsy of his father's original patient. This consisted of an old vascular scar of the corpus striatum on the side opposite the athetosis. The lesion also involved the internal capsule and globus pallidus.

The pathologic basis of athetosis was finally clearly defined in 1911 by Cecile Vogt, who described the changes she found in the striatum in patients with double athetosis, which she called *état marbré* or status marmoratus. The first case she studied involved a patient of our old friend Oppenheim, a 23-year-old girl with strange movements. She carried the clinical diagnosis of hereditary pseudobulbar palsy, because her mother was known to be similarly affected. Careful pathologic study of the brain revealed bilateral atrophy of the striatum. Her second case had been referred by Dr. C. S. Freund of Breslow. In this brain she found foci of myelinated fibers in the striatum that she described as *état marbré*. She believed that both of these patients had a "pure" striatal syndrome:

> We were thus led to construct a syndrome of the corpus striatum, consisting of spasms, more or less accompanied with athetoid movements, rhythmic oscillations, associated movements and spasmodic laughing and crying, without (or almost without) paresis, sensory disturbances or impairments of intelligence—in other words, a pure double athetosis. (*Journal für Psychologie und Neurologie* 18:479–488, 1911)

Nine years later, Cecile Vogt, working with her husband Oskar, described agenesis or imperfect development of the myelin sheaths of the striopallidal fiber systems (status dysmyelinisatus) as another cause of athetosis, and it could be seen with or without torsion dystonia. Although Jakob regarded status marmoratus as the only disorder of the striatum that produced "pure" athetosis, he supported Hammond's original pathoanatomic hypothesis: "My observations show conclusively that athetoid movements in adults are found only in cases in which there are lesions in the pallidum."

Despite the accumulation of evidence of specific pathologic disorders that apparently correlated with clinical syndromes, some clinicians remained skeptical as to the specificity of athetosis. Wilson, in his 1925 Croonian Lectures, discussed this problem:

> Comparing, now, the symptoms of chorea and athetosis, we find the resemblances more impressive than the differences. In respect of the latter, we have seen that chronic movement is discrete and rapid, while athetoid movement is slow and confluent. But this difference is more apparent than real; athetoid action is slow largely because it is confluent, and, on the other hand, confluent chorea results in slowing of the spontaneous movements. Besides, in some athetosis a degree of discreteness and quickness is observable. In respect of resemblance, in each the type of motor derangement is complex, elaborate, and specialized; changeableness and variability of movement is a prominent trait (i.e., absence of essential repetitiveness); the law of reciprocal innervation is at fault in athetosis and in confluent chorea equally; the movements, caricatures though they are in athetosis more than in chorea, have the appearance none the less in the case of the former of being subjectively purposeful—as for grasping or relinquishing an object, etc.—though they are objectively purposeless. ("Disorders of Motility and Muscle Tone with Special Reference to the Corpus Striatum," *Lancet* 2:215–291, 1925)

Over the last 55 years the status of athetosis as a distinct pathophysiological entity or group of entities has gained increasing acceptance. It is now generally believed that Hammond was right that athetosis is a distinct pattern of involuntary movements that can be distinguished from chorea. Athetosis as characterized by increases and decreases of tone in irregular sequences in antagonist muscle groups and slow involuntary movements involving chiefly, not but exclusively, the distal appendicular musculature. As Hammond had suggested but not proved, because he had studied such patients only during life, hemiathetosis usually develops after hemiparesis, as a consequence of necrotizing cerebrovascular lesions that involve the contralateral striatum.

Double athetosis is, of course, a separate disease that usually begins in early infancy, and in almost half the cases there is a history at birth of trauma or anoxia. Double athetosis is most frequently due to bilateral status marmoratus (état marbré) of the striatum, but it can also result from bilateral necrotizing cerebrovascular lesions in the striatum. In rare instances double athetosis may result from bilateral status dysmyelinisatus of the globus pallidus or from bilateral localized destruction in the globus pallidus.

Time and increased information have added more and more support to Hammond's clinically based conclusions about athetosis. Hammond's reason for localizing the lesion contralateral to the striatum was probably the association between athetosis and hemiplegia. At the time of publication of the findings in his two cases it was believed that hemiplegia was due to a lesion of the striatum, which was accepted as the origin of the motor system. Such reasoning may diminish our impression of Hammond's pathophysiological insight, but it does nothing to lessen our respect for his clinical acumen.

William Alexander Hammond was born in Annapolis, Maryland, August 28, 1828, the son of Dr. John W. Hammond of Anne Arundel County. His father's family had been early settlers in Maryland and had originally held large grants from the crown and from Lord Baltimore. Hammond's mother, Sarah Pinkney, traced her descent from a Norman family that had accompanied William the Conqueror. The family name is recorded on the roll of Battle Abbey.

When William was 5 years old the Hammond family moved to Harrisburg, Pennsylvania, where William was educated at an academy. Little is known of Hammond's early life, except that he entered the University of the City of New York at the age of 16, and at the age of 20 he received his M. D. degree. After graduation he interned for a year at Pennsylvania Hospital in Philadelphia. As soon as he completed his internship, Hammond passed the examination of the medical board held in New York on July 29, 1849, and entered the U. S. Army medical service with a rank of assistant surgeon.

The next 10 years of Hammond's life were for the most part spent at various frontier posts in New Mexico, Kansas, Florida, and Michigan. During this time he participated in numerous Indian campaigns, and on one campaign he was the medical director for a large force fighting the Sioux.

His long sojourn in the army stationed at frontier outposts under medically primitive conditions was interrupted by an extended leave that he spent in Europe. Whereas the primary purpose of his European tour was an intensive study of military hospitals, it is probable that Hammond also took advantage of this opportunity to study at various European medical centers. It is possible that he first became interested in neurology at this time. Neurology was just emerging as an independent field and was receiving attention from many leading physicians in the medical centers of the Continent. A visitor to any of these centers could easily have been drawn into neurology, a field that could hardly have been said to exist in contemporary America. On his return he was stationed in Florida and then at West Point.

In spite of his many military activities, Hammond found time to engage in serious and productive scientific investigations, primarily in physiology and physiological chemistry. Although he was truly isolated from any great medical center, Hammond was able to pursue original research, often using himself as the subject of his experiments. By the age of 30 he had published six articles and books, including "Experimental Research Relative to the Nutritive Value and Physiological Effects of Albumin, Starch and Gum, When Singly and Exclusively Used as a Food." This study was awarded the American Medical Association prize in 1857. In this study Hammond left us a self-description:

> I am 28½ years of age, 6 feet 2 inches in height, and measure 38½ inches around the most prominent part of the chest. My weight during the last three years had ranged from 215 to 230 pounds. My habit of body is rather full, temperament sanguinonervous. I am of sedentary habits, rarely taking much physical exercise, unless with some specific object in view other than exercise. I have never indulged freely in alcoholic liquors and very seldom use them now: tobacco I do not use in any form.

During this time he became a close friend of the other founding father of American neurology, Silas Weir Mitchell (1829–1914). Weir Mitchell at this time was already interested in physiology and neurology. In 1859 these two young investigators collaborated in an extensive report on experiments with corroval and vao, two variations of South American arrow poison. This and several other articles were later published by Hammond under the title *Physiological Memoirs*, dedicated to Dr. Mitchell.

Hammond's growing reputation attracted the attention of the authorities of the University of Maryland, and on October 31, 1860, he resigned from the army to take the chair of anatomy and physiology at the medical school in Baltimore. This initial venture into academic medicine started quite well. Hammond's ability as a lecturer, as well as his buoyant personality and limitless energy, promised great success for him as both a teacher and a private practitioner. Other events prevented this, for he had hardly settled into his new life when the Civil War began. The start of the war between the states left Hammond in a difficult position. Baltimore was predominantly a Southern city, and Hammond had very strong Union feelings. Furthermore, he felt great loyalty to the Union army. Shortly after the outbreak of hostilities, Hammond resigned his professorship to return to the army medical service.

Despite his long previous service, regulations at the time required a reexamination, and although Hammond passed this with the highest grade, he lost both the rank he had attained during his former service and his seniority. He was commissioned again as an assistant surgeon.

General Patterson recognized Hammond's experience and knowledge and assigned him to organize hospitals for the army in Hagerstown, Frederick, and Baltimore. Soon after he completed these tasks, General Rosecrans requested an experienced officer, and Hammond was ordered to Rosecrans's headquarters at Wheeling, West Virginia. Once he was there the general made him medical inspector for all camps and hospitals under his command. This assignment gave Hammond an opportunity to demonstrate both his considerable knowledge of hospital needs and his administrative ability.

The army medical service at this time was in a bad state. When the war broke out in 1861, the small standing Union army of 15,000 men was unprepared and was at first unable to cope with a war on this almost unprecedented scale. The army, and almost all of its branches, was commanded by venerable veterans of the War of 1812, now either hopelessly antiquated or nearly senile or both. The medical department was more completely fossilized than other departments. The surgeon general, who at one time had been an able man, was in his dotage, and his principal assistants, having stagnated in a peacetime system, were incapable of carrying out the considerable changes necessitated by war. As slaves to bureaucratic order and army tradition, they were deaf to all entreaties for sweeping reorganization and preparations for war. To critics, the principal occupation of the surgeon general seemed to be merely to sign his name to papers that required that ceremony before they could be admitted to eternal rest in the pigeonholes of the bureau. The deficiencies of the department were apparent to many outsiders. In an attempt to solve this problem, the secretary of war formed a civilian organization, the Sanitary Commission, which was to inquire into and advise him on sanitary conditions in the army. This commission was originally charged with securing information on the needs of the army and giving advice to the medical bureau. Soon after it began its work, it became obvious to the Sanitary Commission that the army medical bureau, as then constituted, was incompetent to carry out its assignment.

The problem was, of course, easier recognized than solved, because the real solution was not within the province of the commission. But the members of the commission were not easily thwarted. They realized that strong action would be required to overthrow the entrenched elders of the bureau, who had both rank and seniority, the two keys to power in the army. Their report was a scathing condemnation of the system:

> It is criminal weakness to intrust such responsibilities...to a self-satisfied, supercilious, bigoted blockhead, merely because he is the oldest of the old messroom doctors of the frontier guard of the country. He knows nothing and does nothing, and is capable of knowing nothing and doing nothing, but quibble about matters of form and precedent.

General McClellan, commander of the Army of the Potomac, was in agreement with the need for radical reform of the medical bureau. Early in 1862 he summoned Dr. Bellows, head of the Sanitary Commission, and asked him to draft a bill for reorganization of the medical bureau. The bill was prepared and endorsed by McClellan and the assistant secretary of war, Thomas A. Scott. At the suggestion of President Lincoln, a strong supporter of the needed reorganization, the bill was introduced by Senator Wilson. Bellows, the author of the bill, described the reform in no uncertain terms: "It strikes at all the senility and incompetence in the Bureau and puts about eight first-class men, selected from the whole medical staff, into control and management of affairs." The principal aim of the new plan was to establish an "administrative and inspectorial" department, which had not previously existed. The bill was quickly pushed through Congress by pressure from the commission and other forces and was signed into law by the president on April 18, 1862.

By this time, Hammond, who was young, vigorous, imaginative, and outspoken, to say the least, had come to the notice of the Sanitary Commission. Hammond's accomplishments were significant. Jonathan Letterman, using data supplied by Hammond and undoubtedly gathered by Hammond during his prolonged leave in Europe, had built the first adequate pavilion hospital at Parkersburg. This was the first U.S. Army hospital with sufficient space and air flow to ensure reasonable sanitary conditions. At the same time, General Rosecrans devised the ambulance that was to be used generally throughout the war. Again, both Letterman and Hammond, with his knowledge of European and especially French military ambulances, had a hand in this project. Hammond's ability in organizing and administering hospitals had also been outstanding.

Finally the reorganization became law, and Surgeon General Finlay resigned. There were numerous candidates senior in rank and age to the 34-year-old Hammond for the vacant office, including one favored by Secretary of War Stanton. Hammond, however, was the choice of the Sanitary Commission. As always in such situations, factors other than ability were important. Stanton wanted his candidate. The commission wanted its candidate. Neither side would yield easily. Some time elapsed before the appointment was finally made, and in the end the commission proved more insistent, or at least more stubborn. These circumstances created an unfortunate situation that could only breed animosities, frustrations, and difficulties.

The appointment of this brash upstart with neither rank (he was only an assistant surgeon) nor seniority (his original tour of duty didn't count under the regulations of the day) obviously brought no joy to the elders of the medical corps. It may be well imagined that those, who had ruled by seniority from the beginning, recognized that they had lost the battle and yielded the title and authority to the new surgeon general, but they had not yet lost the war. In the tradition of passive-aggressive bureaucrats throughout the ages, they knew that their war was far from over. They kept a low profile, seemingly supporting the new order, but all the time they were increasing their seniority and rank, whetting their long knives in preparation for the next major battle. Hammond was as welcome as a Bolshevik to the Romanoffs. History records few deposed royal families that did not dream of returning to power.

Hammond was permitted to select his own assistant surgeon general, and against advice he chose R. C. Wood, an officer popular in Washington social circles, who, having failed to secure the senior position, despite considerable influence, had requested the subordinate post. Doubtless Hammond hoped that this appointment would placate the senior officers over whom he had been promoted. The gesture was futile, of course, and Wood had the good sense to resign within a few months. He was replaced by Dr. J. S. Smith, who became a loyal aide and lifelong friend of Hammond.

On taking office, Surgeon General Hammond found a medical department designed for an army of 15,000 men, but the department would have to meet the requirements of an army of a million or more men. There were eight clerks in the surgeon general's office, and the work was sadly in arrears. Within 2 months the number of clerks had been increased to 60, and this was subsequently increased further to meet increasing demands. Complete reorganization of all departments was required, but from the beginning Hammond was hampered in his efforts. The positions of inspectorships of the hospitals and camps were of utmost importance to the success of his reorganization program. The surgeon general submitted a list of recommendations for these positions to the secretary of war, with Jonathan Letterman named as his choice for inspector general. Four of the inspectors requested by the surgeon general were appointed. The remainder of the positions were given to political appointees. Worst of all, Letterman's nomination was not among those approved, but Hammond later named him medical director of the Army of the Potomac.

C. J. Stillé, in his *History of the Sanitary Commission* (1867), wrote:

> At the very onset, therefore, were the plans of the Surgeon General for the improvement of the service crippled by a refusal to provide him with the means which he deemed necessary to carry them into execution.
> This controversy unfortunately was the cause, or at least the beginning, of a want of cordiality between the Secretary of War and the head of the Medical Bureau, the effect of which is clearly traceable in every part of the history of Dr. Hammond's administration.

Immediately after taking office, Surgeon General Hammond attempted to implement many needed reforms for the welfare of patients. The supply list was vastly enlarged. For the first time, hospital clothing was routinely provided to all patients. Such clothing was essential for men brought in from the filth of days and weeks in the field. A new, more complete system for sick and wounded reports was established. These proved invaluable in the preparation of *The Medical and Surgical History of the War of the Rebellion*, which was finally published in 1870 and was instantly acclaimed the most valuable publication on military medicine of the time. Rudolf Virchow (1871) described these volumes in the following terms: "Whoever takes in hand and examines these comprehensive publications will continually have his astonishment excited anew by the riches of the experience, purchased at so dear a price, which is there recorded." Hammond himself had formulated the original design for this projected 6-volume set.

Hammond recognized the importance of preserving medical reports and specimens for future study. He proposed the establishment of an army medical museum to ensure the accumulation and protection of such material, and he directed all officers to "collect and forward anatomical specimens, surgical and medical, and projectiles and foreign bodies removed and other items that might prove of interest in the study of military medicine and surgery."

The overwhelming need for more and better hospitals was self-evident. Hammond studied the requirements and established a definite program for the erection of adequate facilities. Firmly convinced that proper ventilation would decrease the mortality from disease, he recommended that all new hospitals follow the example of the pavilion hospital built by Letterman in Parkersburg. This structure, based on Hammond's own ideas, assured ample light and air. Hammond was also ahead of his time in recognizing the value of specialized wards and even hospitals to allow for better care of particular types of problems, but also to make the study of particular conditions possible. In two of the large Philadelphia hospitals, wards were set apart for the study and treatment of injuries to the peripheral nerves and the central nervous system. Later, Surgeon General Hammond set up a 400-bed neurologic hospital in Turner's Lane in Philadelphia that was given over to Weir Mitchell, William W. Keen, and George R. Morehouse. The detailed notes that were kept concerning the epilepsies, choreas, nerve injuries, amputations, and palsies formed the basis of their subsequent clinical reports.

The best-known outgrowth of this hospital was the classic *Gunshot Wounds and Other Injuries of Nerves* by S. Weir Mitchell, George R. Morehouse, and William W. Keen, which was published in 1864. This brief book contained only 164 pages and no illustrations. Its greatness rests on its masterful descriptions of nerve injuries, which were simply and thoroughly delineated. Without Hammond's decision to create a specialized hospital, this study could not have been carried out anywhere else nearly as successfully. Mitchell later expanded his experiences into a monograph, *Injuries of the Nerves and Their Consequences* (1872).

In these books, Mitchell was the first to describe causalgia. He gave the first distinct accounts of ascending neuritis, traumatic neurosis, and the treatment of neuritis, as well as other descriptions that have become part and parcel of modern neurology. *Reflex Paralysis*, published in 1864 by Mitchell, Keen, and Morehouse, described paralyses resulting from wounds in remote regions of the body. This, again, was a direct result of their work in America's first neurologic unit. The great American neurophysiologist and medical historian John S. Fulton considered these works milestones in the history of American neurology and clinical medicine.

The successful reorganization of the evacuation system designed by Letterman as medical director of the Army of the Potomac was due in large part to the surgeon general's strong support. It is obvious that both men must have been familiar with Larrey's description of his organization of the French army's medical services during the Napoleonic campaigns. The excellence of Letterman's plan was evident almost immediately. After the second battle of Bull Run (June 29–30, 1862), the wounded of Pope's army lay for a week on the field with inadequate attention. Letterman assumed the medical directorship on July 1, 1862; by August 2 his plans were formulated, and a general order was effected. At Antietam (September 17, 1862), all the wounded had been gathered under shelter within 24 hours.

Surgeon John H. Brinton, who accompanied Hammond to Fredericksburg after the great battle, left us a picture of the surgeon general in action. Hammond did not just sit behind his desk and think.

> I think I then saw him at his best, before his troubles came upon him. Big, burly, and genial; proud of his position in the Army; full of professional feeling,

and anxious to develop good feeling in the Medical Corps, he looked and acted the Surgeon General. He took great interest in the cases and insisted on operating himself. . . . He was well pleased with the medical arrangements.

In order to ensure a medical service of high caliber, Hammond raised the standards for acceptance of physicians into the army and reorganized the board of examiners.

Hammond's vision for the medical corps was projected far beyond his own era. The soundness of his planning is evident in the lasting influence of those reforms he was able to accomplish, as well as the reforms that were blocked during his own administration but were carried out by later surgeons general. These included (1) the establishment of permanent army hospitals, (2) the establishment of an ambulance corps, (3) the establishment of the army medical museum, now the Armed Forces Institute of Pathology, (4) the founding of an army medical school, finally accomplished 100 years later, and (5) the establishment of a permanent hospital research institute in Washington, D.C.

Of all the orders initiated by Hammond, the one that removed calomel from the supply table probably caused the greatest furor. Hammond issued this order after inspections of several hospitals had indicated that the use of calomel had been pushed to excess, with the result that there were frequent cases of mercurial gangrene. In 1863 calomel and tartar emetic were taken off the supply table. The protests were loud and angry, but the order stood. The drug could, of course, be obtained by special requisition when actually needed according to the therapeutic dictates of the day.

Despite the obstacles placed in his path, within a little over a year Hammond brought order out of chaos and laid the foundation for the present army medical service. Although he was quite busy obtaining adequate personnel supplies, and even hospitals, somehow he found time at night to write a comprehensive book on military hygiene, to prepare a manual for military surgeons, and to edit the reports of the Sanitary Commission. He also had Assistant Surgeon Woodward prepare a manual for hospital stewards. Taking advantage of youth, ambition, energy, and enthusiasm, he put life into what had been a moribund department. Not the least of his actions was the selection of Letterman, who devised and put into efffective operation the ambulance system, field supply system, and field hospital system used in all the armies throughout the war. Letterman also instituted a system of corps inspectors and prepared questionnaires and instructions for the inspectors. Those instructions closed with these words: "The prevention of disease is the highest object of medical science." A radical view in 1862.

All of this was not accomplished without stepping on a lot of toes. And Hammond, who often struck people as an arrogant and pompous individual, was neither careful whose toes he stepped on nor apologetic afterward. His relationship with Secretary of War Stanton, who had wanted someone else appointed surgeon general, started badly and continued to deteriorate. Hammond described their original meeting as follows:

I went to his office and the following conversation took place. His tone and manner were offensive in the extreme. He began with a question as to the Sanitary

Commission, and continued, "I want to tell you that if you have the enterprise, intelligence, and brains to run the Medical Department I will assist you." "Mr. Secretary," replied Hammond, "I am not accustomed to be spoken to in that manner by any person, and I beg that you will address me in more respectful terms." "What do you mean?" he exclaimed. Hammond replied, "I was accustomed in the Army, even with low rank, to be addressed in a respectful manner, and as Surgeon General will certainly permit no less." "Then, Sir, you can leave my office immediately," said Stanton.

There was constant friction between these two. Hammond was bright, indomitable in spirit, and arrogant. Stanton was autocratic, irascible, and unrelenting in his prejudices.

The antagonism between Secretary of War Stanton and Surgeon General Hammond steadily increased in intensity. In July, 1863, Stanton appointed a special commission to examine Hammond's activities. This commission was headed by Andrew J. Reeder, who had long been a personal enemy of Hammond.

In August, Hammond was ordered to Hilton Head, Charleston harbor, and other points in the South and West, with headquarters in New Orleans. He was to report to the secretary of war every 10 days. A few days after his departure from Washington, his assistant, Surgeon J. S. Smith, was ordered to St. Louis, where he found orders reassigning him to New Mexico. Medical Inspector J. K. Barnes was directed to perform the duties of the surgeon general. Hammond completed his inspections, returned to Washington, and was again shunted off, this time to Chattanooga and Nashville. On December 2, 1863, Stanton sent him a letter of reprimand, directed him to make no more purchases, and in fact annulled all his powers as surgeon general.

On December 6, Hammond responded, demanding either a court of inquiry or a court-martial. Both Hammond and his friends were confident that a trial would clear his name and reinstate him. As Brinton afterward remarked, "Court-martials sound well, but often do injustice, especially if packed, or when desirous of pleasing superior authority." In all probability the court was not packed, but no member of it would have been considered for a second as a member of a jury in a civilian trial.

When Hammond demanded trial, he showed little insight into his real position. The prosecuting hand was that of Stanton. Stanton, to whom the judge advocate and every single member of the court, as well as the star witness, were beholden. As secretary of war, Stanton could make or break anyone in the army. As if that were not bad enough, the verdict of the court would go to Stanton's judge advocate general for review and then to Stanton himself for final decision. Lincoln had evidently given Stanton a free hand. The first principles of justice require that the judge not be a party to the dispute, but here judge, witness, jury, reviewer, and court of last resort all were minions of the prosecutor. However honest in motive and intention all the participants may have thought themselves, it is unlikely that they could have given Hammond a fair trial.

It is quite probable that Stanton believed Hammond to be corrupt and that his attacks were not personally motivated. This is easily understood. Stanton found the war office swarming with corruption. Grafters were everywhere. He encountered so many bent on cheating the government that he came to suspect everyone. He was always on guard against crooked contractors and conniving officials. Some of Hammond's purchases may have been suspicious. Yet there is now no reason to doubt Hammond's own statement: "The saving of money was altogether a secondary object. My first duty was to save life."

On July 19, 1864, the court proceeded with Hammond's court-martial. There were two charges of "conduct to the prejudice of good order and military discipline," with 10 specifications, all involving irregular purchases of supplies. These specifications suggested that Hammond had exceeded his authority and that he had engaged in personal corruption with intent to aid others to defraud the government. The third charge, an almost trivial charge of "conduct unbecoming an officer and a gentleman," was based on a personal letter to an army surgeon, George Cooper. Hammond was accused of "willful falsehood."

Overall, three separate classes of offenses were included in the specifications: acts in excess of legal authority, acts involving complicity in fraudulent purchases, and the intentional false statement. The first was obviously a hair-splitting, technical charge. Because the duty of purchasing was by law given to purveyors, this charge was based on strict interpretation of law that Hammond could not make purchases. In view of the wording of the law, "medical purveyors shall be charged, under the direction of the Surgeon General, with the selection and purchase of medical supplies," this charge seems almost frivolous. The concept that a superior cannot do what a subordinate can do under his direction appeals to neither logic nor common sense. The custom of ordering purveyors to make purchases existed before Hammond entered the service and continued long after he departed from it. Hammond had ample evidence of this, but it was rejected by the court. Hammond even produced an order for purchase, signed by himself and approved by Stanton, dated November 25, 1862, but the court did not allow it to be placed in evidence.

As for the charges of complicity in fraudulent purchases, these ranged from innuendo to outright deceit. One of the charges for which there was no direct evidence was that excessive quantities of supplies were purchased. This was self-evidently false, if not impossible, in 1862 and 1863. Another was that supplies of poor quality had been purchased by Hammond's direct orders. It was proved in court that none of the supplies were "unfit to be used." It was true that some were not quite up to standard. This will always be the case when, in emergencies, large quantities of supplies are purchased by many agents. The charge that Hammond had in some instances authorized payment of excessive prices for some supplies was similar in nature; although no excessive prices had been paid, some had been higher than others. This has occurred in every war and undoubtedly will continue to occur. Its mere documentation is not proof of fraud. Eliminating these two almost frivolous indictments, there remained the other count against Hammond, that he favored certain dealers. In this regard, two things should be said: first, it was not illegal; second, there may have been good reason for it. Hammond's accusers were perturbed that most of his orders, even those for hospitals near Baltimore, were placed with Philadelphia-based firms, particularly the Wyeth brothers. To them, this smacked of corruption and bribery. But it did not prove that Hammond's motives were personal gain. Philadelphia was unquestionably a better marketplace than Baltimore, and the Wyeth brothers produced a greater variety of supplies and could furnish them more quickly than most of their competitors. It cannot be denied that there were suspicious appearances of favoritism, but there was no direct evidence that this favoritism involved corruption. It was not even charged that Hammond had profited. Here is a sample specification:

> Spec. I. Charge I: That he, Brigadier General William A. Hammond, Surgeon General, U.S. Army, wrongfully and unlawfully contracted for and ordered C.C. Cox, acting Purveyor in Baltimore, to receive blankets of one Wm. A. Stephens, of New York. This done at Washington City on July 17, 1862.

The intimation was that the blankets were of poor quality and were too expensive, but the accusation was not specified and certainly not proved. Any proper court would immediately dismiss this count as indefinite, charging no specific offense. The other charges were similar, in some cases more definite, charging high prices, poor quality, excessive purchases, etc., but all involved matters of opinion, and virtually all specific charges of this sort were refuted. Today they appear to be trumped up. At the worst, Hammond's activities might have been considered to be a little less than circumspect.

Overall, anyone who views the case without prejudice will accept the opinion of the senate committee of 1879: "A careful, unbiased and searching scrutiny of the evidence . . . forces irresistibly the conclusion that the gravamen of all the charges save one (that of falsehood) was either disproved by the defense, abandoned by the prosecution, or eliminated by the findings of the court."

Of the 10 specifications, two were eliminated by the court, and the principal words were eliminated from four others. On the other four counts, the verdict was guilty, without qualification.

The matter of the willful falsehood is easier to reconstruct. The essence of the charge was that when Hammond had written to Cooper that he was transferring him "at the request of Halleck," he was making a false statement. The implication was that Halleck had not requested this transfer. This was a simple issue that anyone could judge. Hammond had sent a personal letter to Cooper containing the following:

> The detail for your relieval [*sic*] from duty went to the Adjutant General's office a few days since. It was with great reluctance, even with pain, that I make this detail. I believe the change would have been made over my head had I not made it myself. This is one reason. The second is even more imperative. Halleck requested it as a particular favor that Murray might be ordered to Philadelphia.

General Halleck was called to testify. He related that he had written the following to Hammond: "Dr. Murray has served long and faithfully with the Army in the field in the West, and he now wishes to be transferred to eastern hospital duty. Please give his case your consideration." Halleck testified further that he had made no other communication with Hammond, in writing or orally, "to the best of my recollection." This alone was insufficient to convict anyone, but more was to follow. Halleck was asked to produce the letter he had received from Murray. He did so the next morning, and it contained these words: "I want to be ordered to duty in Philadelphia, New York, or some point north of these places, Philadelphia would suit me best. If you will send a memorandum to the Surgeon General requesting him to order me to a hospital in Philadelphia it will be done at once." Hammond testified that a day or two later Halleck had asked him to transfer Murray to Philadelphia, not just to any eastern post.

This makes everything clear. Murray had written to Halleck asking to be stationed in Philadelphia. Hammond arranged for him to be stationed there. Hammond stated that this was done at Halleck's request even long before the question was raised. How did this all happen? Either Halleck made the request and forgot it or Hammond was a mind reader. The letter from Murray suggests that Halleck's memory was not reliable. It entirely disposes of Halleck's "best of my recollection" evidence and makes it plain that Hammond's statement to Cooper was the exact truth. How any fair and honest man could convict the surgeon general on this charge is beyond comprehension. The other charges were vague and indefinite, and a confusing mass of evidence might lead to a feeling of foggy doubt. But this charge was plain and simple. The issue was direct, and the evidence was brief and, save on one unimportant point, undisputed. On one point it was clearly disputed. "To the best of my recollection" is the refuge of a hedger, not a condemnation. The verdict of guilty on this charge convicts the court, not Hammond.

As to this charge of falsehood, the senate committee later said the following: "The single charge of which the gravamen was not found wanting by the Court, was in itself trifling, if not frivolous, and certainly insufficient in character and importance to arraign, try, convict, and pronounce sentence thereon, in the manner and form set forth."

When the evidence was finally all in, a verdict was reached in an hour and a half. Hammond was found guilty and dismissed from the army. His dismissal, on August 30, 1864, found him in severely straitened circumstances. He could not afford to move his family from Washington to New York, where he had decided to make his home, until an eminent Philadelphia physician who knew him to be innocent gave him the needed funds. During his first months in New York he wrote articles for newspapers and magazines to support himself.

Following his court-martial, Hammond immediately initiated steps to obtain redress. On Christmas Day, 1864, he petitioned the Senate for an inquiry into the circumstances of his conviction. However, he was not vindicated for 15 years.

With the help of friends he established a practice in neurology, then barely in its infancy. Hammond's first appointment in New York was as lecturer in nervous and mental diseases in the College of Physicians and Surgeons. He rapidly attained prominence as a teacher and clinician, and within 5 years he had become one of the leading neurologists in the country. In 1867 he resigned his position at the college to accept a professorship that had been created for him at Bellevue Hospital Medical College. In 1874 he left Bellevue and became a professor at the University of the City of New York, and he also served on the faculty of the University of Vermont.

Despite his active practice and the demands of his teaching positions, he indulged his investigative mind in a number of research problems. When practicable, he still used himself as the subject. A prolific and facile writer, he produced hundreds of scientific articles, not only on nervous and mental diseases but also on legal medicine, physiology, and a score of other subjects. His studies included the effects of alcohol on the nervous system, abscesses of the liver and their association with hypochondria, and the therapeutic uses of nitroglycerin.

His most famous publication, *A Treatise on Diseases of the Nervous System*, was published in 1871. Although based largely on the lectures of Charcot, it also included Hammond's own personal experiences and his initial description of athetosis. This was the first textbook on nervous diseases published in the United States. It passed through nine editions in the next 25 years and was translated into French, Italian, and Spanish.

The broad range of Hammond's interests and accomplishments is suggested by a sampling of his other scientific works: *On Wakefulness: With an Introductory Chapter on the Physiology of Sleep* (1866), *The Physiology and Pathology of the Cerebellum* (1869), *Spiritualism and Allied Causes and Conditions of the Nervous Derangement* (1876), *A Treatise on Insanity and Its Medical Relations* (1883), *Sexual Impotence in the Male and Female* (1883).

Hammond was also a prominent figure in the field of medical journals. He established the *Quarterly Journal of Psychological Medicine* and *Medicine and Medical Jurisprudence* in 1867 and was its editor for 8 years. He also aided in founding and editing the *New York Medical Journal* and was an associate editor of the *Journal of Nervous and Mental Diseases*.

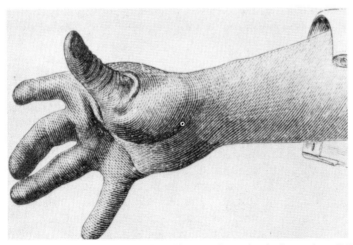

FIG. 1. Original illustration of athetosis from Hammond's textbook of neurology (1871).

One of his most important achievements was his effort to organize the fledgling field of neurology. Initial attempts to form an active neurologic organization in New York began in 1872. There was at that time a group of eminent neurologists in New York, 10 of whom had formed the New York Neurological Society. This society soon became dormant. It was Hammond, with his usual abundance of energy and organizational ability, who put life back into it, issuing the following call to the neurologists of New York:

Dear Sir:

It is contemplated to reorganize the New York Neurological Society (instituted March 1872), and you are respectfully invited to cooperate in this work.

Probably no department of medicine is advancing with greater rapidity than that which relates to the Physiology, Pathology and Therapeutics of the Nervous System. It is not doubted that there are, in this city and its vicinity, many who will take such an interest in this society as to render it of great service to medical science.

Believing you to be of this number, this circular is addressed to you, in the hope that you will become one of the original members.

Should you accede to this proposal, please address a note to that effect, at your earliest convenience, to either of the undersigned.

Due notice will be given of the first meeting of the society.

Respectfully

Your obedient servant,

William A. Hammond, 43 W. 54th Street
Alexander Murray, 23 East 10th Street
J. Marion Sims, 267 Madison Avenue
J. C. Peters, 83 Madison Avenue
Max Hertzog, 48 West 34th Street

Forty-three physicians responded, and the first meeting was held April 6, 1874. At this meeting Dr. Hammond made it clear that the purpose of the meeting was to revive the New York Neurological Society, which for all practical purposes had accomplished nothing in the 2 years of its existence. Apparently all those present agreed with Dr. Hammond, and he was elected president of the reborn society.

This was the first neurological society in America. The Philadelphia Neurological Society was founded in 1884, with Weir Mitchell as its somewhat reluctant president. In contrast, the Neurological Society of London, with Hughlings Jackson as president, was not founded until 1886.

Less than a year after the founding of the New York Neurological Society, Hammond began another effort to organize American neurologists. It was because of his efforts that six of his colleagues, four of them from New York, were stimulated to help in the founding of the American Neurological Association.

By 1878 Hammond had acquired sufficient funds to make another attempt to have his record cleared. He managed to have the matter brought up before Congress, and with but one dissenting vote it was recommended that a senatorial committee should review the evidence and forward their recommendations to the president for final action. Hammond was completely vindicated and was placed on the retired list as a surgeon general, with the rank of brigadier general. Following his vindication, the following editorial appeared in the *Journal of Nervous and Mental Diseases:*

> It certainly cannot be considered other than appropriate, that we should congratulate our eminent co-worker, Dr. Hammond, on his restoration to the high rank he had attained in the medical department of the army of the United States, during the early part of the civil war, and on the completeness of his final vindication from the misdemeanors, which it has been since seen, were so unjustly imputed to him.
>
> Dr. Hammond may have even grave faults, as some have thought, but no one familiar with his history during and since the war, will in candor, withhold a sincere admiration for the courage, industry, indomitable perseverence and elasticity of spirit which he has shown, in the midst of a host of difficulties which would have disheartened, or even crushed an ordinary man.
>
> He has triumphed over them, and has placed himself, in many respects, at the head of his profession in his own country, and has made himself widely and favorably known abroad. All this has been accomplished in a comparatively short period in time, and by his personal exertions, apart from outside aid, and even in spite of hostile opposition.
>
> Dr. Hammond has not yet passed his prime, and retains in full measure his physical and mental powers, and lives in the enjoyment of a notable success, both as a practitioner and author, especially in nervous and mental diseases—in that high and difficult department in medicine, which he was the first among American physicians to occupy in a prominent manner.
>
> May he long live to enjoy the well earned rewards of a successful professional life.

Hammond's private means permitted him to waive the usual retirement income.

In addition to his numerous professional articles and books, Hammond wrote a number of successful novels and even tried his hand at writing plays. In 1867 he published his first novel, *Robert Severne, His Friends and Enemies*, and the next year he arranged for the printing of a 1663 translation of the works of Virgilus, an Italian who lived in England during the reigns of Henry VII and Henry VIII. These works had not previously been printed in the United States. Most of his literary work was done later in his career. Five novels were published between 1884 and 1887. They were typical nineteenth-century romances. In the last decade of his life he became increasingly interested in religion, and his last novel, *The Son of Perdition* (1898), was a historical novel that centered around the life of Christ.

In 1888 Hammond, then 60 years old, retired from his professorship, relinquished his extensive private practice, and returned to Washington, where he opened a sanitarium for the treatment of nervous diseases. He was soon forced to curtail his practice because of heart disease, from which he died on January 5, 1900.

His career after he was dismissed from the army was not devoid of controversy. He believed that cocaine was of value in treating "opium habit" and could be used successfully without inducing any "so called cocaine habit." He had used cocaine successfully in cases of spinal irritation, especially in cases of "cerebral hyperemia." He believed it was useful in melancholia and in hysteria with depression of the spirits. He did not deny that there was a cocaine habit, but he compared it to a coffee habit. He also advocated the use of cocaine in hay fever, but he admitted treatment failures in cases of masturbation. A discussant of his 1886 presentation about cocaine at the New York Neurological Society thanked Hammond for his timely presentation. This discussant recognized the morbid fear of cocaine that was spreading throughout the country and hoped that the words of Dr. Hammond would "allay the prejudice against a most useful remedy." Fortunately, Hammond's influence here was only short-lived.

NOTES

There are three reasonably accessible histories of involuntary movement disorders, each of which reflects the background of its author. F. H. Levy's "Historical Introduction: The Basal Ganglia and Their Diseases" (research publication, *Journal of Nervous and Mental Disease* 21: 1–20, 1942) emphasizes the history of anatomic and pathologic study of the basal ganglia in the nineteenth and twentieth centuries. Francis Schiller's "The Vicissitudes of the Basal Ganglia" (*Bulletin of the History of Medicine* 41:515–539, 1967) provides a scholarly historical approach to the development of our concept of the basal ganglia from ancient times. Andre Barbeau, in his article "The Understanding of Involuntary Movements, An Historical Approach" (*Journal of Nervous Mental Disease* 127:469–489, 1958), blended a clinical approach with biographic sketches of important contributors and a review of pathology and pathophysiology.

A brief sketch of Hammond's life, with emphasis on his literary pursuits, has been written by L. C. McHenry ("Surgeon General William Alexander Hammond," *Military Medicine*, 128:1199–1201, 1963). E. E. Drayton's "William Alexander Hammond" (*Military Surgery*, 199:559–565) gives more details of his army career and later accomplishments. The most complete view of his court-martial is that of L. C. Duncan ("The Days Gone By," *Military Surgery*, 64:98–110, 252–262, 1929). Hammond's role in organizing American neurology is described in B. Stookey's "Historical Background of the Neurological Institute and the Neurological Societies" (*Bulletin of the New York Academy of Medicine* 35:707–729, 1959). Of the various biographies of S. Weir Mitchell, I prefer Richard D. Walter's *S. Weir Mitchell, M. D.—Neurologist* (Springfield, Ill.: Thomas, 1974). Mitchell's work on war injuries is also discussed in D. J. LaFia's "S. Weir Mitchell on Gunshot Wounds and Other Injuries of Nerves" (*Neurology* 5:468–471, 1955). Hammond's views on cocaine are readily found (*Journal of Nervous Mental Disease* 13:754–759, 1886).

Edward Selleck Hare
and
Silas Weir Mitchell
and
The Discovery of Horner's Syndrome

Not to know the events which happened before one's birth is to remain always a boy.

Marcus Tullius Cicero
(106–43 B.C.E.)

Edward Selleck Hare
and
Silas Weir Mitchell
and
The Discovery of Horner's Syndrome

The components of the Horner syndrome (ptosis, miosis, enophthalmos, and alterations in sweating and vasomotor control in the head and neck) and its localizing significance (dysfunction of the cervical sympathetic system) are too well known to deserve lengthy discussion. But the history of the discovery of this disorder is not as well known and deserves retelling, because several individuals other than Johann Friedrich Horner made contributions worth remembering.

François Pourfour du Petit (1664–1741), a noted French surgeon, made the first significant contribution to our understanding of the physiology of the cervical sympathetic system. In 1727, in *Memoires de Mathematique et de Physique* of the Royal Academy of Sciences, he published a detailed account of experiments in which he cut the vagosympathetic nerve trunk in dogs (Fig. 1). Immediately following such surgery, Petit noted "sinking in of the globe, narrowing of the palpebral fissure, injection of the conjuntiva and relaxation of the nictitating membrane." He also observed diminution in the size of the pupil in several experiments, but this may not have been an immediate effect. Petit was careful to distinguish between the respiratory difficulties he observed and attributed to sectioning of the vagus nerve and the effects on the eye, which he believed to be related to paralysis of the sympathetic nerves. The only other significant contribution made during the eighteenth century was a series of experiments by William Cruikshank, who repeated and confirmed Petit's work but made no mention at all of any miosis.

In 1839, John Reid, a noted physiologist from Edinburgh, also studied the functioning of the cervical sympathetic system and concluded that "the contraction of the pupil, the relaxation of the nictitating membrane, and the partial approximation of the eyelids to each other, take place immediately after injury of the sympathetic."

Seven years later, Serafino Biffi, in his doctoral thesis at the University of Pavia, reported that galvanic stimulation of a severed cervical nerve produced dilatation of the miotic pupil. The next year, 1847, Ruete, a professor at the University of Göttingen, in an article entitled "Physiology Applied to Ophthalmology," stated that the pupil becomes wider if the sympathetic nerve is stimulated, but smaller if the sympathetic nerve is paralyzed. He compared these effects with the sympathetic influence on the action of the heart. He also observed that in paralysis of the third nerve the dilated pupil could be made to dilate still further by the use of belladonna. On the basis of these findings, Ruete suggested that there are two types of motor nerves acting on the pupil and that these two types of nerves correspond with the

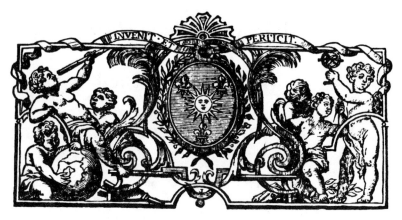

MEMOIRES

DE

MATHEMATIQUE

ET

DE PHYSIQUE,

TIRE'S DES REGISTRES
de l'Academie Royale des Sciences.

De l'Année M. DCCXXVII.

MEMOIRE

dans lequel il eſt démontré que les Nerfs Intercoſtaux
fourniſſent des rameaux qui portent des eſprits
dans les yeux.

Par M. PETIT, Medecin.

J'AY lû au mois de Decembre dernier un Memoire dans
lequel je détermine l'endroit où l'on doit picquer l'œil
pour bien abbattre la Cataracte : j'y remarque une choſe qui
Mem. 1727.   **A**

FIG. 1. Title page of François Pourfour du Petit's *Memoires de Mathematique et de Physique.*

two varieties of muscle fibers known to exist within pupillary muscles. Further, he
inferred that the sympathetic nerves innervate the radial fibers, which produce
dilatation, and that the third nerve supplies the circular fibers, which cause the iris
to contract. This suggestion, when first published by Ruete, was not wholly substantiated experimentally, but eventually it proved to be true.

In 1851 Julius Ludwig Budge and Augustus Waller found that the fibers of the sympathetic system had their origin in the spinal cord. In animal experiments they found that cutting the sympathetic fibers at their origin produced the same effect as cutting the nerve in the neck. Like previous experimenters, they found that cutting the sympathetic nerve in experimental animals caused constriction of the homolateral pupil and that stimulation of the same nerve produced pupillary dilatation. This latter experiment was also performed on the newly decapitated head of a condemned criminal. In these studies Budge and Waller paid particular attention to alterations in the size of the pupil, giving little attention to other effects.

It was left for Claude Bernard, the greatest of all French physiologists, to make the first complete study of all the physiological effects of both sectioning and stimulating the cervical sympathetics. Claude Bernard was born in 1813 in St. Julien, a Rhone village noted primarily for the red wines produced in the area. His father was one of the many winegrowers of the region. Family financial difficulties forced him to cut short his education at the college at Villefranche and become a pharmacist's assistant in nearby Lyon. There, influenced by the growing romantic movement, he became interested in the theater. He wrote *La Rose du Rhone*, a vaudeville comedy that was produced locally with some success, and *Arthur de Bretagne*, a five-act tragedy that was not produced.

Encouraged by his local success, the 21-year-old Bernard took his unproduced tragedy and traveled to Paris, where he showed his work to the great critic Saint-Marc Girardin, who was then a professor at the Sorbonne. Girardin received him kindly and read the manuscript with great care. Although it is traditionally believed that Girardin remarked that Bernard had some merit as a dramatic poet, he in no uncertain terms advised Bernard to pursue literature in his leisure moments and turn to something else as a profession. Because Bernard had already studied pharmacy, Girardin advised him to take up medicine, which he was certain would be more likely to guarantee a livelihood than playwriting. This advice, which Bernard followed, marked the turning point in his career. This well-known story smacks of the romanticism of the era that influenced both scientists and their biographers. Because his financial means were meager, Bernard taught natural history in a girls' school for several years in order to finance a medical education. Finally he entered the College de France, and in 1839 he became an intern under Magendie at the Hotel Dieu in Paris. Two years later he became Magendie's préparateur. In this position it was Bernard's responsibility to prepare all of the experiments, which Magendie then demonstrated to the students. Here Bernard's natural aptitude for experimentation soon became evident. After the third or fourth demonstration, Magendie is said to have told Bernard "You are better than I." Through his day-to-day contact with Magendie, the father of experimental physiology in France, the direction of Bernard's scientific career was determined. Experimental physiology, not the clinical practice of medicine, was for him. He spent many productive years with Magendie, first as an assistant in the senior investigator's experiments and as a collaborator in scientific papers. As the years passed, Bernard began to work on his own problems, write his own papers, and slowly but surely demonstrate that

Magendie's estimate of his ability had been correct. Magendie, although he made great discoveries during his career, often went about his work in a somewhat haphazard fashion. Bernard's approach was very different; his experiments were always rigorously designed, and as little as possible was left to chance.

Bernard's attitude toward scientific investigation is best summed up in his own words:

> Put off your imagination, as you take off your overcoat, when you enter the laboratory; but put it on again, as you do your overcoat, when you leave the laboratory. Before the experiment and between whiles, let your imagination wrap you around; put it right away from you during the experiment itself lest it hinder your observing power.

Bernard's first paper was on the anatomy of the chorda tympani. His second, which was his thesis for the degree of M.D. in 1843, described experiments on intravenous injection of cane sugar. In the first of these he found that cane sugar, when injected into a vein, appears in the urine. In a second experiment he discovered that this does not occur if the sugar is treated with gastric juice prior to being injected. After receiving his degree, he switched his activities from the hospital wards to the laboratory. He never practiced medicine.

Bernard's three most important contributions to physiology were his demonstration of the role played by pancreatic secretions in digestion, his discovery of the glycogenic function of the liver, and his extensive studies of vasomotor function. He also studied carbon monoxide poisoning and found that carbon monoxide displaced oxygen in red blood cells. He investigated curare and, in 1850, showed that it blocks the communication between nerve and muscle, but that the muscle still responds to electrical stimuli.

In 1852 Bernard published two papers in which he gave a detailed report on the effects of sectioning of the cervical sympathetic nerves. He described the following sequelae that resulted from the sectioning: (1) constriction of the pupil and injection of the conjunctiva, (2) retraction of the eyeball into the orbit and relaxation of the nictitating membrane, (3) narrowing of the palpebral aperture, (4) diminution of intraocular tension and progressive diminution in the size of the eyeball, (5) a decrease in the size of the nares, and (6) an increase in temperature over the face on the same side with flushing. With his usual thoroughness, Bernard then went on to show that all six of these conditions were reversed if the peripheral end of the cervical sympathetic nerve was stimulated. He reported that such stimulation resulted in pupil enlargement, opening of the palpebral fissure, forward movement of the eyeball in the orbit, a decrease in circulation, and pallor of the conjunctivae, nares, and ears, which had been red. When he stopped the stimulation, all the phenomena he had described after sectioning of the sympathetic nerve returned.

In 1855 Magandie died and bequeathed his chair of medicine at the College de France to his assistant, who by that time was giving the courses for him. Although Claude Bernard held a professorship of general physiology first at the Sorbonne and later at the Musée d'Histoire Naturelle, his heart always belonged to the College de France, where Magendie and he had worked so long together.

Other honors also came to Bernard. In 1849 he was made a chevalier of the legion of honor. The citation, in glaring error, reads "for his excellent work on the musical properties of the pancreas." In 1861 he was elected to the Academie de Medicine and in 1868 to the Academie Francaise; in 1869 he was made a senator by imperial decree of Napoleon III. However, his personal life was not happy. His marriage was not a success. Even his daughters became estranged from his as a result of his wife's influence. Mme. Bernard had no sympathy with his genius. She was disappointed by the fact that he had not become a successful and wealthy practitioner. Girardin's economic advice had not been fully carried out. Although it was true in the Paris of the Second Empire that it was more profitable to be a physician than a playwrite, the monetary rewards of an M.D. did not extend to include nonclinical academicians such as Bernard.

Bernard died in 1878 at the age of 64. Pasteur said of him that he was not a physiologist but physiology itself. His birthplace, an old farmhouse in his beloved St. Julien, is now preserved as a national monument. It is on a quiet hill surrounded by vineyards. Claude Bernard had returned there each summer late in his life to reflect on his experiments and their significance.

At the time of death, Bernard had been studying fermentation, and after his death his notes on these experiments were published. Among other things, these notes contained the sentence "Alcohol is formed by a soluble ferment outside of life." This statement greatly irritated Pasteur, who maintained there could be no fermentation without life. A bitter scientific controversy followed. Pasteur and his followers maintained that fermentation involved living organisms, whereas those who pursued the work of Bernard believed that fermentation was simply a chemical reaction. In 1895, 17 years after Bernard's death, Buchner separated a substance from yeast cells that, when added to sugar, caused fermentation, with the production of alcohol and carbon dioxide.

Of course, both sides were right in this scientific debate. Pasteur was in one sense correct in maintaining that fermentation required life (a cell or an enzyme produced by such a cell), and Bernard was right in his belief that fermentation is a chemical reaction that can occur without living cells. Had Bernard been able to consider these last studies in the quiet of St. Julien, much of the vicious controversy of the next 20 years might well have been avoided.

According to tradition, the next contribution to an understanding of the Horner syndrome was made by the Swiss ophthalmologist Johann Friedrich Horner, whose name is now linked to the syndrome of cervical sympathetic dysfunction. Horner was born in Zurich in 1831, the son of a well-regarded physician. Johann learned the classics, mathematics, and natural history at a primary school in Zurich, and after his military service he entered the University of Zurich in 1849. There he pursued his interest in natural science and then medicine. Among his various teachers, it was apparently the great experimental physiologist Carl Ludwig who had the most significant influence on Horner. In 1854 Horner received his doctor's degree from the University of Zurich with highest honors. His thesis dealt with the purely orthopedic problem of the curvature of the vertebral column in the sitting position.

Following graduation he spent the next year traveling to several major medical centers to broaden his education. His stops included first Munich and then Vienna. Horner attended lectures on a great variety of clinical subjects, but he was more attracted to ophthalmology than to the other specialties. In Vienna, Friedrich von Jaeger, then in the twilight of his long career, showed Horner the first volume of the new *Archiv für Ophthalmologie*, published by his former student, Albrecht von Graefe. Horner was obviously impressed and immediately went to Berlin to study with von Graefe.

Albrecht von Graefe (1828–1870) is often described as the creator of modern ophthalmology. A native of Berlin and the son of an eminent military surgeon, von Graefe had studied medicine at Berlin, where he received his degree in 1847. He then studied at Prague, where he came under the influence of Ferdinand Arlt, professor of ophthalmology, and decided to become an opthalmologist. Following further study in Paris, Vienna (where he came into contact with von Jaeger), and London, he returned to Berlin in 1850 and began practice as an eye specialist. The development of the ophthalmoscope by Helmholtz in 1851 was greeted enthusiastically by von Graefe, who was the first ophthalmologist to exploit this valuable tool. Using this instrument he was able to diagnose sudden loss of vision from embolism of the retinal artery (1859); he pointed out the importance of optic retinitis in diagnosis, and he differentiated between functional and organic loss of vision. He introduced the operation of iridectomy for treatment of iritis, iridochoroiditis, and glaucoma. He employed linear extraction in operations for cataract, and he noted the lid malfunction in exophthalmic goiter (von Graefe's sign). He founded the *Archiv für Ophthalmologie*, in which he described most of his important discoveries. This journal led its field for more than half a century.

Von Graefe became associate professor of opthalmology at Berlin in 1857 and professor in 1886, and he directed the most productive ophthalmology clinic of his time. Physicians like Horner came to him from all over the world seeking instruction, and patients came in even greater numbers to obtain his advice and treatment. He died in 1870 when only 42 years of age.

In 1859 the New Sydenham Society printed a translation, by T. Windsor, of von Graefe's discussion of the role of increased intraocular pressure in glaucoma and his use of iridectomy to relieve the pressure:

> Now when I compared the general appearance of the glaucomatous inflammation with that of other internal inflammation, for example, of the common irido-choroiditis, it seemed to me that all the characteristic symptoms tended to one point—increase of the intra-ocular pressure.
>
> The hardness of the glaucomatous globe has been remarked from the earliest periods of ophthalmology. Since no change in the sclerotic, capable of explaining the altered resistance of the globe, can be justly admitted, it must be founded on the more complete filling of the globe with fluid.
>
> Supported by these facts and considerations, I considered myself perfectly justified in performing iridectomy in glaucoma; for I knew the favorable action of the operation on the condition of the choroid in regard to its circulation; and everything seemed to favour the opinion that the operation probably possessed a

physiological, and certainly, in many cases, a therapeutical pressure-diminishing action. The first trials were extremely uncertain, for I had no fixed principles, either in regard to the choice of cases or the manner of making the trial. I first employed this method in June 1856, and from that time have continued to it, especially in the cases which I have already described as acute glaucoma.

Von Graefe was not the only ophthalmologist working in Berlin when Horner arrived there. Helmholtz was there, as was the great French ophthalmologist Donders, who did so much to develop perimetry. But it was to von Graefe that Horner went, and von Graefe welcomed him as a student and friend.

From Berlin, Horner went to Paris, where he had a highly profitable and stimulating period of study at the eye clinic of Desmares. While in Paris he published his first contribution to ophthalmology, a paper that outlined those manifestations of systemic disease that could be seen and diagnosed by use of the ophthalmoscope.

Following his travels, Horner returned to Zurich, where, after a few years of practice in general medicine, he began a specialized practice in ophthalmology. In 1862 he was named professor of ophthalmology at the University of Zurich. He continued in active practice until his premature death in 1886 at the age of 55.

Horner made many contributions to the developing field of ophthalmology, including work on keratitis, glaucoma, and cataracts. His most important contribution, or at least his best-known contribution, was a short paper entitled "Ueber eine Form von Ptosis" ("About a Type of Ptosis"). This paper was published in 1869, and in it he described the syndrome that now bears his name. This description has been translated by John Fulton:

> Many of my colleagues are familiar with chronic cases of incomplete ptosis in adults, which lack the usual accompanying signs of oculomotor paralysis but exhibit the remarkable sign of a myosis of the pupil on the same side. This clinical picture was not new to me when at the end of last November a 40 year old woman presented with these symptoms. Less than one week later I saw them again in a woman of about the same age, but it was not possible for me to obtain such crucial information for the elucidation of the ptosis in this case as it was in the first. I may be permitted, therefore, to report here on the first case.
>
> Frau Anna Brandli, aged 40, a healthy-looking peasant woman of medium size, seems to have suffered since adolescence from generalized headache which in the course of recent years had rather diminished in frequency and intensity.
>
> Six weeks after her last confinement, which occurred a year ago, she noticed a slight drooping of her right upper eyelid, which increased very gradually and for about three months had remained constant. The upper lid covers the right cornea to the upper edge of the pupil; the lid is not loose or wrinkled but somewhat sunken into the orbit and is still capable of movement; it is neither injected nor swollen. The upper convex furrows on the right side of the forehead indicate that the frontalis muscle is working as a substitute (for the levator palpebrae superioris).
>
> The pupil of the right eye is considerably more constricted than that of the left, but reacts to light; the globe has sunk inward very slightly and repeated determinations showed that it was somewhat less firm than the left. Both eyes are emmetropic, and have normal visual acuity and early presbyopia.
>
> During the clinical discussion of the case, the right side of her face became red and warm, the color and heat increasing in intensity under our observation, while the left side remained pale and cool. The right side seemed turgid and rounded,

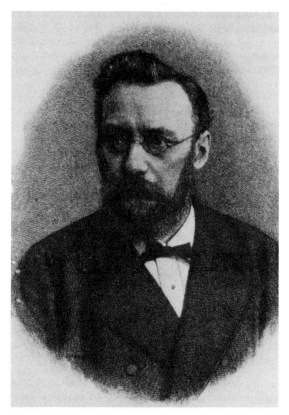

FIG. 2. Contemporary engraving of Johann Friedrich Horner that appeared as the frontispiece to his *Ein Lebensbild geschrieben von ihm Selbst, erganst von Dr. Landolt* (1887).

the left more sunken and angular; the one perfectly dry; the other moist. The boundary of the redness and warmth was exactly in the midline.

The patient told us that the right side had never perspired, and that the flushed feeling, and also the ptosis, had only developed in the course of the last year. The redness of the right side of the forehead and cheek was said to be present in the evening as a rule but was also brought on more or less markedly at other times by any emotion.

(Horner, with two associates, then documented the decrease in temperature in the right cheek and to a lesser degree in the right axilla.)

Two points necessitate the conclusion that the vasomotor disturbance involves not only the trigeminal area, but also that of the fibers of the cervical sympathetic: first, the slight but distinct variation in temperature in the axillae, secondly, and more important, the small size of the right pupil.

The latter symptom prompted some investigations concerning the action of atropine and calabar. When equal quantities of atropine were instilled into each conjunctival sac the right pupil enlarged slowly and irregularly; after twenty minutes it had not yet reached the size of the left, but remained more constricted and oval, even though more drops were put into the right eye.

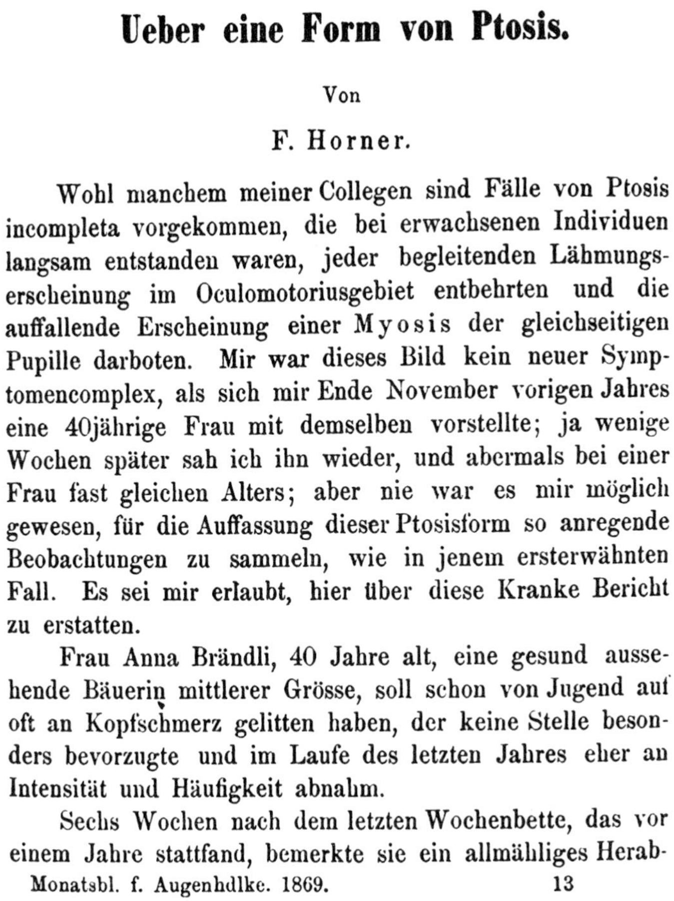

Ueber eine Form von Ptosis.

Von

F. Horner.

Wohl manchem meiner Collegen sind Fälle von Ptosis incompleta vorgekommen, die bei erwachsenen Individuen langsam entstanden waren, jeder begleitenden Lähmungs- erscheinung im Oculomotoriusgebiet entbehrten und die auffallende Erscheinung einer M y o s i s der gleichseitigen Pupille darboten. Mir war dieses Bild kein neuer Symp- tomencomplex, als sich mir Ende November vorigen Jahres eine 40jährige Frau mit demselben vorstellte; ja wenige Wochen später sah ich ihn wieder, und abermals bei einer Frau fast gleichen Alters; aber nie war es mir möglich gewesen, für die Auffassung dieser Ptosisform so anregende Beobachtungen zu sammeln, wie in jenem ersterwähnten Fall. Es sei mir erlaubt, hier über diese Kranke Bericht zu erstatten.

Frau Anna Brändli, 40 Jahre alt, eine gesund ausse- hende Bäuerin mittlerer Grösse, soll schon von Jugend auf oft an Kopfschmerz gelitten haben, der keine Stelle beson- ders bevorzugte und im Laufe des letzten Jahres eher an Intensität und Häufigkeit abnahm.

Sechs Wochen nach dem letzten Wochenbette, das vor einem Jahre stattfand, bemerkte sie ein allmähliges Herab-

Monatsbl. f. Augenhdlke. 1869.   13

FIG. 3.   First page of Horner's original article.

When, twenty-four hours after the atropine, equal quantities of calabar were put into the conjunctival sac of each eye, one noticed after ten minutes a marked constriction on the right, and after half an hour almost maximal myosis, while on the left the action of the atropine still continued, and it was only after a half hour that an insignificant decrease of the effect of the atropine was apparent.

(Calabar is an extract of the dark brown poisonous seed of a woody vine, *Physostigma venenosum*, native to tropical Africa and containing physostigmine. In 1863 Argyll Robertson, whose name is now associated with pupillary abnormalities he described in certain patients with syphilitic involvement of the spinal cord, first described the properties of the calabar bean as an ophthalmologic agent.)

I have already mentioned that the right globe always appeared somewhat softer, but the difference was slight, even if constant. Measurements were made with a Dor tonometer, which is adequate for such comparisons. This difference in tension suggested comparing also the diameter of the retinal vessels. When observed during the stage of elevation of temperature, the veins of the right retina appeared wider and more tortuous than the left, a difference which did not exist when the whole right side was cool, as it was, for example, when the opthalmoscopic examination was made in the early morning. However, the differences found were so slight that only through repeated examinations by several investigators can the results be securely established.

It is not too much to assert that his experiment with belladonna and calabar speaks for the dual control of the movements of the iris in man; differences in color and caliber of the vessels of the irides have not been found, and therefore it is most probabale that we are dealing with right dilator paralysis.

The explanation of the difference in the tension relations of the globe is as yet a matter of personal opinion, since the various functional components of what the anatomist calls the trigeminus cannot yet be accurately distinguished by experimentation.

Let us now turn to the question of the causation of the ptosis. I believe that nobody who had seen all the foregoing symptoms, would be surprised at my considering this ptosis, which comes on gradually but remains incomplete, to be a paralysis of the musculus palpebrae superioris supplied by the sympathetic nerve (H. Muller, Harling), and the appearance of the upper lid as part and parcel of the whole symptom-complex. It would thus appear to be the opposite of the condition in exophthalmic goiter in which the upper lid is drawn upward, or better, into the orbit, which by von Graefe and Remak is described as due to the stimulation of the muscle fibers of the lid.

In this brief paper Horner carefully documented all of the manifestations of dysfunction of the cervical sympathetic system, and he was able to relate the signs and symptoms to cervical sympathetic dysfunction. He was able to do this because of his familiarity with the experimental work of Claude Bernard, Budge, and others. However, he made no diagnosis as to cause and presented no pathologic proof that he was correct. Today it is unlikely that a single report such as this would be accepted for publication. Yet this brief paper describing an undiagnosed patient has been hailed as the first clinical description of this disorder, and the author's name has been forever linked with the disorder.

But was Horner the first clinician to describe Horner's syndrome? In 1838 Edward Selleck Hare (1812–1838), a house surgeon of the Staffordshire County General Infirmary, wrote a short paper that appeared the day after his untimely death. In this paper Hare described a patient with a rapidly growing tumor arising on the left side of the neck that gave rise to symptoms of compression of the brachial plexus and miosis and ptosis on the left. This paper appeared in the *London Medical Gazette*:

TUMOR INVOLVING CERTAIN NERVES

To the Editor of the Medical Gazette

Sir,

If your are of the opinion that the points connected with physiology and pathology in the following case, render it worthy of a place in your very valuable publication, I shall be much obliged to you to give it insertion.

I am, sir, your obedient servant,

EDW. SELLECK HARE, M.R.C.S.

House-Surgeon to the Stafford County General Infirmary.
September 11, 1838.

Thomas Willetts, aged 40, married, of an unhealthy complexion, was admitted to the Infirmary, under the care of Dr. Knight, on the 8th of last June. He had been attacked a month before with pain, tingling and numbness along the course of the ulnar nerve of the left arm, which was most severe at the elbow, where there had also been some swelling and redness. There was, besides, pain through the left shoulder, extending across the chest to the opposite side, and upwards to the left eye and teeth of that side; also a sense of pulsation in different parts of the body, and sleepless nights. The tongue was clean, appetite good, no cough, or physical sign of pulmonary disease, and the secretions were all natural.

After a careful examination, the only cause that could be discovered to account for his symptoms was a small tumor, situated in the "inferior triangular space," on the left side of the neck, which it was possible might be producing some pressure on the origins of the nerves going to form the brachial plexus: the pulse at the wrist was equal to that of the other arm. The tumor, however, did not appear to be more than an enlarged gland, and the disease was supposed to be of a scrofulous nature.

In addition to the foregoing symptoms, the pupil of the left eye became contracted; and the levator palpebrae ceased to perform its office, the general irritability increased almost to mania, and the bowels became very torpid. In about three weeks after his admission, the pains and distressing sensations appeared to be increased, the pulse had become quicker, there were signs of debility, with numbness and coldness of the lower extremities; also by this time the tumor of the neck had become more extensive, and possessed a remarkable degree of hardness.

(The tumor progressed, and the patient died August 26.)

Post-mortem inspection.—The examination of the body was begun twenty-eight hours after death: it was now greatly emaciated. There was aedema to a small extent in the legs and left arm.

The brain and spinal prolongation and their investing membranes were carefully examined, but no disease of any kind was detected. The optic nerves were of the same size and firmness; that portion of the medulla spinalis which swells into the cauda equina was particularly firm; there was little or no fluid in the great cavity of the arachnoid, not a large quantity in the lateral ventricles, and that in the spinal canal inconsiderable.

Dissection of the tumor.—After dissecting back the skin and platisma, from the left side of the neck, the superficial cervical fascia was found to be unusually dead, and the cellular tissue about it infiltrated with serous fluid. It being removed, the tumor presented its irregular surface, and was found to possess the hardness of scirrhus. Some considerable veins passed into its substance, and it extended under the sterno-cleido-mastoideus and trapezius, raising on its surface the omohyoid, sterno-hyoid, and thyroid; which however, were not implicated in the disease. After the removal of these, the tumor was seen to extend upwards as far as the origin of the brachial plexus. The carotid artery, internal jugular vein, and pneumo-gastric nerve, passed into its substance; the first remaining pervious, the two last lost and transformed into the diseased structure, as were also the phrenic nerve, and further down the sympathetic, with its lowest cervical ganglion. The jugular vein above the tumor was atrophied, and the pneumo-gastric nerve was aedematous. The scirrhous mass extending under the clavical, the latter was removed, and the following were its further relations:—The subclavian artery and vein passed into its substance, that portion of the anterior scalenus which separates the artery and vein, and nearly the whole of the muscle, being included in the disease, and undistinguishable. Both the artery and vein were pervious, but the latter was filled with a coagulum of a deep red colour. The tumor extended inwards as far as the trachea and arteria innominata, and downwards behind the left vena innominata, and downwards behind the left vena innominata and subclavian and carotid arteries, as far as the aorta, impinging upon it at the junctions of its arch with the descending portion. The thoracic duct passed into and was lost in the disease, as also were the recurrent laryngeal nerve, and the veins accompanying the branches of the subclavian artery,—the branches of that artery themselves passing through the tumor without being converted into its nature. The tumor lay upon the brachial plexus, being firmly attached to the spine at the origin of the third and fourth nerves of the plexus, both which were inseparable from it.

Upon cutting into the anterior surface of the scirrhus, watery pus escaped, and the surrounding cellular tissue was aedematous. The carcinomatous mass extended itself in company with the last cervical and first dorsal nerves between the transverse processes, and into the intervertegral foramina as far as to the dura mater, which appeared beginning to be implicated; but the canal was perfect, and the appearance of the theca of the medulla not at all altered. There was no appearance of carcinoma in any other part of the body.

Observation.—The case seems to be interesting as an instance of glandular scirrhus in the male. The connection of the disease with the distress and paralysis along the course of the ulnar and median nerves is obvious, and is evidence in confirmation of the assertion that the nerves can be traced through the plexus to the last cervical and first dorsal nerve, which I believe Boyer denies. The paralysis of the levator palpebrae, which receives a branch from the third pair; the contraction of the pupil; the pain of the teeth; the distressing sensation across the upper parts of the chest; the paraplegia; the sense of pulsation in various parts of the body; and the maniacal disturbance of the mind, cannot, I apprehend, be referred to any direct communication between the structural disease and these several affections, but rather they must be regarded as an instance of that remote sympathy which is found to exist between distant parts of the same individual, and is most frequently displayed in persons of a nervous temperament. The aedema of the arm might possibly depend on the existence, during life, of the coagulum found in the sub-clavian vein; but the swelling of the elbow, which occurred at a much earlier date, could scarcely be supposed to depend on any impediment to the circulation at that period, and is interesting as showing how pain and irritation of the nerves of a part, existing only sympathetically with a distant cause, may lead to structural alteration in such part, and is parallel to what occurs in hysterical females, of which I have seen many examples. The stoppage of the thoracic duct with much emaciation, perhaps is parallel to maintenance of "enbonpoint" by hysterical patients, with the most complete anorexia for very long periods. The length of time during which the patient was bedridden, and the degree of emaciation and debility, taken together, were not sufficient to account, of themselves, for the sloughs over the sacrum and hip, which probably owed their existence to the paralysis of the nerves of animal life; and the fact tends to demonstrate the influence of this part of the economy over the nutritive functions.

It is clear from the preceding that Hare did publish a reasonably complete clinical description of Horner's syndrome, 31 years before Horner's paper; but, unlike Horner, he was unaware of the physiology that would explain the signs and symptoms. Hare had no notion at all that there was any relationship between the tumor involvement of the cervical sympathetic chain and the ipsilateral miosis and ptosis. The differences between the two papers are striking. Writing in 1869, Horner was aware of the function of the cervical sympathetic nerve, but he did not know the cause of the dysfunction in his patient, nor did he prove that the cervical sympathetic nerve was involved. Hare, writing 31 years earlier, knew the cause and even knew that the tumor involved the cervical sympathetic nerve, but he was unaware of any relationship between the cervical sympathetic system and the ipsilateral eye. Had he but read his Petit, the syndrome might be named after Hare rather than Horner. But, alas, he had not, and his attempt to classify the syndrome in his patient as a remote effect of carcinoma does not appear to be valid.

Hare was born in Staffordshire, the son of a farmer, and at age 20 (1832) entered the University College in London. He did well there and became a member of the Royal College of Surgeons in 1834. He became house surgeon at the Stafford County Infirmary in 1837 and died the next year of typhoid fever. He was buried at St. Mary's Church, Stafford, and the following inscription was placed on his tombstone:

> *EDWARD SELLECK HARE, M.R.C.S.*
> *House Surgeon to the Stafford County Infirmary*
> *Died 28th Sept. 1838 aged 26 years.*
>
> *Distinguished in his short career, as well*
> *By scientific acquirement and*
> *Professional knowledge,*
> *As by exemplary Christian deportment;*
> *And early falling a sacrifice in the*
> *Fearless discharge of professional duty;*
> *This tablet is erected by his*
> *Official connections in the Infirmary and other friends;*
> *In testimony of their high sense*
> *Of his public and private worth,*
> *Who*
> *"By the grace of God, was what*
> *He was."*

Because Hare was unaware that the cervical sympathetic nerves were related to the ptosis and miosis of his patient, it is probably better that his name is not attached to the syndrome of cervical sympathetic dysfunction. The same cannot be said of the three American clinicians.

In 1864, a full 5 years before Horner published his single case report, there appeared the following description of a 24-year-old soldier with a gunshot wound to the right side of his neck:

> The pupil of the right eye is very small, that of the left eye is unusually large. There is a slight, but very distinct ptosis of the right eye and its outer angle appears as though it were dropped a little lower than the inner angle. The ball of the right eye looks smaller than that of the left. This appearance existed, whether the eye was open or closed and gave the organ the look of being tilted out of the usual position. The conjunctiva of the right eye is somewhat redder than that of the left

and the pupil of the right eye is somewhat deformed, oval rather than round . . . the right eye having become myopic.

These authors also observed that when their patient walked around in warm weather, "his face became distinctly flushed on the right side only and pale on the left." When resting, no difference was found in the temperatures of the two sides of the mouth or ear. Five months later the patient was dismissed from medical care to return to his military duties. At that time, nearly all of his peculiar symptoms had disappeared, and the clinical study came to an end. In discussing the case, the authors stressed the point that all the observed signs were due to a lesion of the cervical sympathetic nerve. Unlike Hare, they pointed out that the symptoms they described were similar to the effects of cutting the cervical sympathetic nerve in animal experiments. They also discussed all other possibilities that might be contributing factors to such symptoms, such as spinal concussion. But their final conclusion was as follows: "We ourselves are of the opinion that this case was a case of injury of the sympathetic nerve and if so it is probably the only one recorded." This case report was placed by the authors in a chapter entitled "Wound of the Sympathetic Nerve," and in the introduction to the case report, Weir Mitchell, Morehouse, and Keen wrote the following: "During our long connection with this hospital we have encountered one single case of lesion of the sympathetic nerve." It seems clear that these authors described Horner's syndrome 5 years before Horner did. Like Horner, they understood its pathophysiology, but their study was more complete because they knew the cause of the lesion in their patient.

The preceding description was published in *Gunshot Wounds and Other Injuries of Nerves*, by S. Weir Mitchell, G. R. Morehouse, and W. W. Keen. This 164-page book is considered to be the first classic of American neurology. It was a by-product of Surgeon General William A. Hammond's determination that individual classes of war injuries be segregated to different hospitals, each of which would have a staff oriented to those particular problems. One of the problems that Hammond believed required such specialization was traumatic nervous disorders. The location of this hospital was Turner's Lane in Philadelphia, and Silas Weir Mitchell, an old friend and collaborator of Surgeon General Hammond, was assigned there. Weir Mitchell described this work at Turner's Lane military hospital in these words:

> With Keen and Surgeon Alden as Surgeon-in-Chief and by special order relieved of much of the time dilling, red-tape business, we set to work. Both Morehouse and I had at that time increasing general practice, but a morning visit to the hospital disposed of the routine work and about three p.m., or later, we went back . . . worked on at note-taking often as late as twelve or one at night and when we got through, walked home, talking over our cases. Usually the work took four or five hours and we did it all in person. The late hours came two or three times a week and usually followed a inflow of cases of injuries to nerves after some serious battle. I have worked with many men since, but never with men who took more delight to repay opportunity with labor . . . the opportunity was indeed unique and we knew it. The cases were of amazing interest. Here at the time were eighty epileptics and every kind of nerve wound, palsies, choreas, stump disorders. I sometimes wonder how we stood it.

Weir Mitchell, Morehouse, and Keen published their study of war injuries involving nerves in 1864. In their introduction they described the source of their patient material:

> The great bulk of our patients has consisted of men who have been shifted from one hospital to another, and whose cases have been the despair of their surgical attendants. As the wounded of each period of the war have been cured, discharged, invalided, or died, every large hospital has had left among the wards two or three or more strange instances of wounds of nerves. Most of them presented phenomena which are rarely seen, and which were naturally foreign to the observation even of those surgeons whose experience was the most extensive and complete. Nowhere were these cases described at length in the text-books, and, except in a single untranslated French book, their treatment was passed over in silence; while even in the volume in question but a limited class of nerve lesions was discussed. In the great monographs on military surgery, this defect is still so complete, that wounds of nerves are there related as curiosities and as matters for despair, than with any view to their full clinical study and systematic treatment.
>
> Our materials for this study consist of about one hundred and twenty cases, all of which have been carefully reported in our note books during the past year. No labor has been spared in making these clinical histories as perfect and full as possible. Those only who have devoted themselves to similar studies will be able to appreciate the amount of time and care which have been thus expended. We indulge the hope that we shall leave on record a very faithful clinical study of nerve injuries, and that we shall have done something at least toward lessening the inevitable calamities of warfare.

This book not only contained the first description of Horner's syndrome but also took the first systematic approach to injuries of the central and peripheral nervous systems. As such, it is a landmark in the development of clinical neurology. The most famous of all the clinical descriptions in this book is that of "burning pain," which Weir Mitchell later called causalgia.

> We have some doubt as to whether this form of pain ever originates at the moment of the wounding; but we have been so informed as regards two or three cases. Certain it is that as a rule, the burning arises later, but almost always during the healing of the wound. Of the special cause which provokes it, we know nothing, except that it has sometimes followed the transfer of pathological changes from a wounded nerve to unwounded nerves, and has then been felt in their distribution, so that we do not need a direct wound to bring it about.
>
> The seat of the burning pain is very various; but it never attacks the trunk, rarely the arm or thigh, and not often the forearm or leg. Its favorite site is the foot or hand. In these parts it is to be found more often where the nutritive skin changes are met with; that is to say, on the palm of the hand, or palmar face of the fingers, and on the dorsum of the foot; scarcely ever on the sole of the foot or the back of the hand. Where it first existed in the whole foot or hand, it always remained last in the parts above referred to, as its favorite seat.
>
> The great mass of sufferers described the pain as superficial, but others said it was also in the joints, and deep in the palm. If it lasted long, it was referred finally to the skin alone.
>
> Its intensity varies from the most trivial burning to a state of torture, which can hardly be credited, but which reacts on the whole economy, until the general health is seriously affected.

The part itself is not alone subject to an intense burning sensation, but becomes exquisitely hyperaesthetic, so that a touch or a tap of the finger increases the pain. Exposure to the air is avoided by the patient with a care which seems absurd, and most of the bad cases keep the hand constantly wet, finding relief in the moisture rather than in the coolness of the application. Two of these sufferers carried a bottle and a sponge, and never permitted the part to become dry for a moment.

As the pain increases, the general sympathy becomes more marked. The temper changes and grows irritable, the face becomes anxious, and has a look of weariness and suffering. The sleep is restless, and the constitutional condition, reacting on the wounded limb, exasperates the hyperaesthetic state, so that the rattling of a newspaper, a breath of air, another's step across the ward, the vibrations caused by a military band, or the shock of the feet in walking, gave rise to increase of pain. At last the patient grows hysterical, if we may use the only term which covers the facts. He walks carefully, carries the limb tenderly with the sound hand, is tremulous, nervous, and has all kinds of expedients for lessening his pain. In two cases at least, the skin of the entire body became hyperaesthetic when dry, and the men found some ease from pouring water into their boots. They said, when questioned, that it made walking hurt less; but how or why, unless by diminishing vibration, we cannot explain. One of these men went so far as to wet the sound hand when he was obliged to touch the other, and insisted that the observer should also wet his hand before touching him, complaining that dry touch always exasperated his pain.

Since the above was written, the advance of General Grant has filled our wards with recent nerve wounds, among whom are several cases of burning. One of them is a mere lad, whose repetition of all the peculiar and singular statements of older sufferers is a strong confirmation of the truth of their complaints. As the present case had never been in a hospital before, and as when he entered our wards there were not marked cases of burning, he could have had no previous chance of acquiring knowledge sufficient to enable him to repeat in detail every singularity of our former cases.

The authors gave the following explanation of this new disorder:

> The rational of the production of this form of pain was at first sought for among reflex phenomena. It then seemed to us probable that a traumatic irritation existing in some part of a nerve trunk was simply referred by the mind to the extreme distribution of this nerve, agreeable to the well-known law of the reference of sensations. Further study led us to suspect that the irritation of a nerve at the point of wound, might give rise to changes in the circulation and nutrition of parts in its distribution, and that these alterations might be themselves of a pain-producing nature. The following considerations tend to strengthen the view, that the immediate cause of burning pain lies in the part where the burning is felt.
>
> If the burning were a referred sensation, it would sometimes be met with in cases of complete division of nerves, and, therefore, in parts devoid of tactile sensation. But we have encountered no such cases, and, on the other hand, the burning pain is often accompanied with hyperaesthesia, while motion and touch may remain unaltered. Is it not probable that the depraved nutrition, often so marked in the congested, denuded, and altered skin, may give rise to a disease of the ultimate fibres of the sensitive nerves? Just such a pain comes when we attack the cutis with irritants; and, let us add, that the agents which help these cases of burning are those addressed to the spot where the pain is felt, and not to the cicatrix.

This book was widely read, and its description of causalgia continues to be quoted today. Why has their description of cervical sympathetic paralysis been overlooked?

There is no simple answer to this question. Perhaps their short description of Horner's syndrome was simply overshadowed by their more significant contributions.

Who were Weir Mitchell, Morehouse, and Keen? Silas Weir Mitchell was one of the founders of American Neurology. He needs little introduction. He was born in Philadelphia in 1829 to a distinguished family that included several physicians over three generations. After a desultory preparatory education, Mitchell was admitted to the college department of the University of Pennsylvania in the class graduating in 1848; he left because of ill health a year before graduation. He graduated in medicine at the Jefferson Medical College in 1850 and spent a year (1851–1852) in Paris, where he came in contact with Claude Bernard, the physiologist, who greatly influenced the course of his future work. As a student of Bernard in 1852, he would have been fully aware of Bernard's work on the functioning of the cervical sympathetic system. On his return from Europe at the age of 23 years, he became his father's assistant and practiced general medicine and, later, neurology.

The Civil War had a profound impact on his life and work. At the outbreak he was 30 years of age, vigorous and eager to serve. He lived in the midst of a recruiting area and saw the thousands march through Philadelphia toward the front. He had a place in the work of the Sanitary Commission and of the army hospitals; early in the war he was appointed acting assistant surgeon. In two of the large military hospitals of Philadelphia, wards were set apart for him, for the study and treatment of injuries of the peripheral nerves and of the central nervous system. In 1863 a large hospital was established at Turner's Lane, a Philadelphia suburb, where several hundred patients were available for study by Mitchell and his colleagues, Morehouse and Keen.

Following the Civil War he returned to the private practice of neurology in Philadelphia. In 1875 he introduced the "rest cure" for nervous disorders, and for the next 20 years he continued to make significant contributions to clinical neurology. He was a renowned lecturer, and his *Clinical Lecture on Nervous Disease* (1897) was widely read.

His list of honors is truly impressive. It includes numerous honorary degrees and memberships in various honorary societies in many countries, including Germany, France, United Kingdom, Sweden, Italy, and others. During the last 30 years of his life he spent much of his time writing not scientific papers but novels, poetry, short stories, essays, and even plays. He wrote 19 novels, many of which were based on his own experiences in the Civil War. Only one of these, *In War Time*, which originally appeared in 1884, remains in print. His breadth of accomplishments is such that during his lifetime he was considered to be the most versatile American since Franklin. He died in Philadelphia in 1914.

Mitchell's associate, George Read Morehouse (1829–1905), was born at Mount Holly, New Jersey, March 25, 1829. His family history is interesting. At some time before the war for independence, Andrew Morehouse emigrated from the north of England to the colony of New York. He later served as a colonel during the American Revolution. His son Abraham, apparently a man of means, seems to have been led into the wild land speculation that during Washington's terms in office ruined so many. He bought vast tracts of coal lands in Virgina and Pennsylvania; in Louisiana he acquired an entire parish, the territorial equivalent of a county. This parish still bears his name. After his death, these possessions were lost because of nonpayment of taxes. His only child, Doctor G. R. Morehouse's father, was finally left in comparative poverty, but in time he became the rector of the Protestant Episcopal Church of St. Andrew, Mount Holly, New Jersey, and retained this charge for 46 years. Dr. Morehouse's mother was Martha Read, a granddaughter of Joseph Read, former attorney for the crown in the Province of New Jersey. George Morehouse graduated from Princeton College in 1848 with high honors. In September of that year he matriculated at the University of Pennsylvania. He left it at the close of one term for the Jefferson Medical College and was graduated from there in 1850. In the following year he received an M.A. from Princeton.

Finally he also received an M.D. from the University of Pennsylvania. In the early 1850s he settled in Philadelphia and began life as a general practitioner. Aside from his collaboration with Weir Mitchell, he wrote little. Weir Mitchell described their relationship in these terms:

> Early in the Civil War Dr. Morehouse served in the Filbert Street Hospital as assistant surgeon under contract. When the Hospital for Nervous Diseases was organized I asked to have him as my colleague. Then Dr. William W. Keen joined us and we remained in useful co-partnership of labor up to 1865.
>
> During our long service he operated often and had the skillful hand, the ready decision of the moment, and the courage which might have made him a surgeon of distinction. I recall two instances of his capacity. In one desperate case of paralysis he removed through the mouth a bullet which had lodged in the cervical vertebrae. The patient recovered. I saw him trephine the skull and open a cerebral abscess, the first case I believe on record unless one by Detmold preceded it.

His skill as a surgeon resulted in a large and successful private practice. He died of renal disease on November 12, 1905.

William Williams Keen (1837–1932), third member of this Civil War neurologic team, was born in Philadelphia. He was graduated from Brown University in 1859 and from the Jefferson Medical College in 1862. He at once entered the army as acting assistant surgeon and soon became generally known because of his association with Mitchell and Morehouse in their notable work and publications on nerve injuries. After the war he spent 2 years studying in Europe.

In 1866 he returned to Philadelphia, began the practice of medicine, and soon acquired teaching positions. For 9 years he lectured on pathological anatomy at the Jefferson Medical College. During the same period he conducted the Philadelphia School of Anatomy, in which he had been preceded by many distinguished surgeons. From 1876 to 1889 he was professor of artistic anatomy at the Philadelphia Academy of Fine Arts, and from 1884 to 1889 he was professor of surgery at the Women's

Medical College. During the period between 1866 and 1889 Kenn became known in the world of surgery through his contributions to the literature.

In 1889 he was elected one of the professors of surgery at the Jefferson Medical College. He gave up his other hospital and college positions and devoted himself to teaching, to his surgical service in the Jefferson Hospital, and to writing. He became America's first "brain surgeon" and soon gained and held preeminence in this field of surgery. He died in 1932 at the age of 95.

Historical priority notwithstanding, the syndrome of cervical sympathetic dysfunction is usually called Horner's syndrome by clinicians. In France, of course, the French contribution is also recalled, and the hyphenated eponym Claude Bernard-Horner syndrome is often used. At one time, physiologists used the name Budge's phenomenon. No one has ever seen fit to honor Weir Mitchell, Morehouse, and Keen or the unknown criminal studied by Budge.

NOTES

The great American neurophysiologist and medical historian John Fulton did much to help unravel the true history of the Horner syndrome and the roles played by both Horner and Hare in its discovery. His discussion ("Horner and the Syndrome of Paralysis of the Cervical Sympathetic"), as well as his complete translation of Horner's "Ueber eine Form von Ptosis," can be found in *Archives of Surgery* (18:2025–2039, 1929). In another article, "Edward Selleck Hare and the Syndrome of Paralysis of the Cervical Sympathetic" (*Proceedings of the Royal Society of Medicine*, 23:152–159, 1929), he described Edward Hare's life and his one report, "Tumor involving Certain Nerves." Fulton apparently was unaware of the description published by Mitchell, Morehouse, and Keen. Bruno Kisch, in an article entitled "Horner's Syndrome: An American Discovery" (*Bulletin of the History of Medicine*, 25:284–288, 1957), corrected this oversight.

A Plague of Mice

They had not been many days in Attica before the plague first broke out among the Athenians. Previously attacks of the plague had been reported from many other places in the neighbourhood of Lemnos and elsewhere, but there was not record of the disease being so virulent anywhere else or causing so many deaths as it did in Athens. At the beginning the doctors were quite incapable of treating the disease because of their ignorance of the right methods. In fact mortality among the doctors was the highest of all, since they came more frequently in contact with the sick. Nor was any other human art or science of any help at all. Equally useless were prayers made in the temples, consultation of oracles, and so forth; indeed, in the end people were so overcome by their suffering that they paid no further attention to such things.

> Thucydides, Introduction to his
> description of the plaque which struck
> Athens in 430 B.C.E.

A Plague of Mice

Ten times Moses went unto Pharaoh. Ten times Moses told Pharaoh that the Lord God of Israel said "Let my people go." But Pharaoh knew not the Lord God of Israel. Ten times Pharaoh, with hardened heart, refused to let the people of Israel go. Ten times the Lord God of Israel inflicted plaques on the Pharaoh and his people, each plague more terrible than the previous one:

Blood,
Frogs,
Lice,
Wild beasts,
Pestilence,
Boils,
Hail,
Locusts,
Darkness,
The slaying of the first born.

Modern readers of the book of Exodus use the term *plague* in the more limited sense than did Moses. To us, a plague is an infectious disease, a sudden but widespread one with a high mortality rate. But even in an age when the news of every sort of natural disaster is instantly flashed before our eyes this three thousand year old list of calamities seems complete. What else could the Lord God of Israel have visited upon the Pharaoh and his people? This question would have had an obvious answer to anyone living at an earlier time, in an agricultural economy. They would have immediately known that one of the most common afflictions which has continued episodical attacks upon mankind and his food supply was not on this list, that God had spared the Egyptians one rather simple common devastation. The missing form of recurrent disaster, a type which is rarely if ever even acknowledged by historians or theologians, is the prosaic plague of the field mouse.

Each such plague of field mice, or their first cousins, the voles and lemmings, is an impressive culmination of their insurgent subterranean activity. In each a picture of devastation breaks like a tidal wave upon the crops. Of all man's efforts, all of his vigilance and care are not enough. His land is inundated by myriads of small, swift, flitting forms that infest the ground and devour everything. Every remedy is tried: poison, plowing, fumigation, trenches, floods, fires, and prayers. None seems to work, and the destruction goes on. Charles Gerard, a nineteenth-century French naturalist and lawyer, wrote about an outbreak of field mice that he had witnessed as a boy in his native Alsace in 1822: "It was a living and hideous scourging of the earth, which appeared perforated all over like a sieve."

In this same work, "Essai d'une Faune historique des mammiféres sauvage de l'Alsace," published in 1871, Gerard also wrote of detailed description of these all too often ubiquitous assailants. According to Gerard, the vole wears a livery entirely suitable to the surroundings. Its coat is a short jacket of russet over a dull brown waistcoat, and its clothing is completed by small white accessories. This is altogether a fine costume for a life in the fields. The vole makes up for any lack of skill or size by a virtually unquenchable thirst for activity. It takes no notice of the sun, but works morning, noon, and night. With such incessant activity, and a taste for almost every kind of crop, it is not surprising that the vole makes a success of its life.

The resources of nature, it seems, are not equal to the task of supporting continued demands of such a degree. All food resources become exhausted, and then as suddenly as it began, the plague abates, and for some years the land is allowed to recover. Each plague has followed somewhat the same identical course. Every country of Europe and Asia has witnessed these disasters which have either been more common or better recorded in Gerard's native France. The most, if not all of the bigger outbreaks, have found their way into that country's annals. Such plagues are records for 1271, 1278–79, 1366, 1378, 1468, 1538, 1539, 1617–19, 1652, 1719, 1742, 1794, 1801–2, 1818, 1822, 1856, and 1861. There is no regular pattern in these occurrences; they average about three to a century, or one to a generation. Some came at closer intervals. But they have been so spaced out that few of the people living at any time during the last 700 years can have failed to experience at least one great plague of this kind.

The field mouse involved in these plagues in Europe is the Continental vole (*Microtus arvalis*), known in France as *campagnol*, in Germany as *Feldmaus*, in Holland as *Veldmuis*, in Italy as *Topo campagnolo*, and in Denmark as *Sydmarkmus* (souther field mouse).

There are other subsidiary species that have ravaged these countries, but seldom with the thoroughness and rapacity of *M. arvalis*. One such species is *M. agrestis*, the only species on the mainland of Great Britain and in Norway. In these countries, occasional plagues brought by these mice have taken their place with the best, or worst, that voles have achieved.

It is clear that the Lord God of Israel was well aware of this form of natural disaster, and it has been suggested that the earlies field mouse plague was recorded in the Bible, not, of course, as one of the 10 plagues visited on the hard-hearted Pharaoh and his people, but as part of the punishment of the Philistines at Ashdod for carrying off the Ark of the Covenant following their defeat of the Israelites.

The tradtional Masoretic text (1 Samuel 6) introduced the plague without reference to field mice: "But the hand of the Lord was heavy upon them of Ashdod and He destroyed them and smote them with emerods, even Ashdod and the borders thereof." The Vulgate and the Septuagint give a somewhat different introduction: "Mice were generated and boiled over the towns and fields in the midst of that region and there was a confusion of great death in the land." (1 Kings 6).

The Philistines called for their priests and diviners to learn how to abort the devastation. The priests told them that the ark must be returned, but not empty. They must send a guilt offering; then, and only then, would they be healed. According to the texts, the guilt offering was to be "five golden emerods, and five golden mice, according to the number of the Lords of the Philistines; for one plague was on you all, and on your lords." They placed the golden emerods and the images of the "mice that mar the land" in the ark and carried them beyond their frontiers. And thus the ark was returned with five golden mice, and the plague abated.

Today, the plague of the Philistines, as it is now called, is generally considered to have been the first description of bubonic plague. The emerods are depicted as being buboes, and the golden mice are not a specific reference to field mice or voles but a more generic reference to small flea-bearing rodents. Elton, however, in his history of visitations of rodents, *Voles, Mice and Lemmings* (Oxford: Clarendon Press, 1942), was of the opinion that this was the first example of a plague of field mice:

> In spite of sweeping changes in God and circumstances, Authority has for several thousand years continued to act in much the same way, even to the present day. The Bible story is, if you like, a parable. The affair runs always along a similar course. Voles multiply. Destruction reigns. There is dismay, followed by outcry, and demands to Authority. Authority remembers its experts or appoints some: they ought to know. The experts advise a Cure. The Cure can be almost anything: golden mice, holy water from Mecca, a Government Commission, a culture of bacteria, poison, prayers denunciatory or tactful, a new god, a trap, a Pied Piper. *The Cures have only one thing in common: with a little patience they always work.* They have never been known entirely to fail. Likewise they have never been known to prevent the next outbreak. For the cycle of abundance and scarcity has a rhythm of its own, and the Cures are applied just when the plague of voles is going to abate through its own loss of momentum.

Aristotle, in his *Historia Animalium*, described the rapid proliferation and equally perplexing disappearance of these small rodents:

> The phenomena of generation in regard to the mouse are the most astonishing both for the number of the young and for the rapidity of recurrence in the births. . . . The rate of propagation of field mice in country places, and the destruction that they cause, are beyond all telling. In many places their number is so incalculable that but very little of the corn-crop is left to the farmer; and so rapid is their mode of proceeding that sometimes a small farmer will one day observe that it is time for reaping, and on the following morning, when he takes his reapers afield, he finds his entire crop devoured. Their disappearance is unaccountable: in a few days not a mouse will be there to be seen. And yet in the time before these few days men fail to keep down their numbers by fumigating and unearthing them, or by regularly hunting them and turning in swine upon them; for pigs, by the way, turn up the mouse-holes by rooting with their snouts. Foxes also hunt them, and the wild ferrets in particular destroy them; but they make no way against the prolific qualities of the animal and the rapidity of its breeding. When they are superabundant, nothing succeeds in thinning them down except for rain; but after heavy rains they disappear rapidly.

This description, written in the fourth century before the common era, was so accurate and comprehensive that the next 2,400 years have added very little to an understanding of the factors that control the mouse population. Aristotle's brief paragraph contains most of the components of the problem of natural fluctuations.

Most other ancient writers were concerned primarily with the human disasters that resulted from such fluctuations. Some accounts, of course, were mere anecdotes, embroidered with fanciful stories about mice. The frequent occurrences of these tales do show that plagues of mice were well known to the ancient chroniclers.

One of the best of the ancient stories was recorded for us by Herodotus. In Second Kings (probably c. 686 B.C.E.), King Sennacherib of Assyria and his multitudes were besieging Jerusalem: "And it came to pass that night, that the angel of the Lord went out, and smote in the camp of the Assyrians an hundred fourscore and five thousand: and when they arose early in the morning, behold, they were all dead corpses. So Sennacherib king of Assyria departed and went and returned and dwelt at Nineveh." The Bible does not give any more details, but Herodotus, who never missed a change to retell a good story, does. According to his version, the disaster was brought about by field mice that poured in on the soldiers, devoured the soldiers' quivers, bowstrings, and even the leather or rope handles of their shields, so that the next day while attempting to retreat, they were attacked and overwhelmed, with great loss of life. Herodotus is believed to have seen a statue of the Egyptian Pharaoh Sethon, who was a contemporary and bitter enemy of Sennacherib. This statue, in the temple of Vulcan, showed Sethon with a mouse in his hand to commemorate the defeat of his Assyrian rival.

Many historians now believe that the Assyrians may have died from bubonic plague or some other rodent-carried disease and that the story telescopes these happenings into a single night. The defeat of the Assyrians by God-sent mice may not be a strictly historical event. Vole plagues may not even occur near Jerusalem, where the Assyrian cohorts camped, although there are other rodents in the neighborhood that might have played a part. True or not, accurate or not (and historical truth and accuracy as we understand them were not part of Herodotus's approach to history), this story does show the respect one ancient historian had for field mice. Herodotus was not alone. Respect for the lowly field mouse was both widespread and well deserved. It is manifested in documents from throughout the Mediterranean, the Aegean, and beyond. Diodorus Siculus described one plague: "In Italy it came to pass that the field-mice in the plains appeared in such numbers that the inhabitants were driven away." Strabo, in his geography, wrote that Spain, the land of the Iberians, was often the site of devastating waves of pestilence because of the great numbers of mice that lived there. When the Roman army was in Cantabria, there was an explosion in the mouse population; there were shortages of everything, especially grain, and famine ensued. People engaged in catching the mice were generously rewarded for delivering mice to the authorities, but this had little effect.

According to Pliny, Theophrastus had reported that mice on the island of Gyaros multiplied to such an extent that they drove all of the human population off the island. Pliny, always a naturalist, recorded his first-hand observations on mouse plagues. He noted that the numbers of mice increased until the harvest was utterly destroyed and that they then diminished remarkably rapidly. He was bewildered by this, because no one knew how it was that such a multitude died, and he recorded that "neither are dead ones found, nor is there anyone who has dug up a mouse in winter in his field." The Troas, the region of the legendary city of Troy, was subject to these invasions, and the inhabitants of that country had even at times been driven out by the mice. "Their appearance takes place in dry seasons. It is said that when they are about to die, a worm is generated in their heads."

Aelian has preserved for us another ancient story from farther East. He credits one Amyntas as the original sourse for a description of mouse plague in the region of the Caspian Sea. According to this story, mice in this region at certain times appeared in prodigious numbers. They filled the rivers, which in that region are rather formidable in size and swiftness. They ate all the grain in the fields, climbed the trees and devoured the fruit, and even nibbled the branches. The Caspians defended themselves against these invasions of mice by raising birds of prey. When the mice invaded, the Caspian tribesmen would counterattack by releasing their birds, which would cover the sky like dark clouds and devour the mice.

Had the plagues ended with the fall of the Roman Empire and the end of the ancient world, one could look on them as a topic for detached study by historians. But they did not, and the practical problem remains what it has been for several thousand years: how to anticipate and deal with each new plague, or, better yet, how to stop such multiplication and control the mouse population. The basic problem remains the same, whether the mouse plague is destroying alfalfa in Nevada, spruce trees in Scotland, peach orchards in Italy, or wheat fields in Canada or Thessaly.

In the last 100 years, first bacteriologists and then microbiologists have entered the field and attempted to control such plagues with pestilences of their own. None other than Louis Pasteur (1822–1895) was the first scientist to suggest the use of an infectious agent to control economically harmful animal populations. Because of his numberous contributions to modern medical microbiology, it is often forgotten that Pasteur was not a physician and that for most of his career he studied industrial problems, not medical problems. Pasteur is best remembered for such advances as his discovery that infectious agents could be attenuated and that such attenuated agents could still produce immunity, findings that had application in his development of the first successful rabies vaccine. Although this was the crowing achievement of his career and was a prime example of his ability to begin an investigation with a simple hypothesis and progress past numerous obstacles to a clear-cut solution, it was one of the few medical acheivements of his investigative life. His successful career was based on work in which he applied his knowledge of bacteria to the making of vinegar, to the prevention of wine spoilage, to improving French beers, and to eradicating diseases of silkworms, an accomplishment that saved the French silk industry.

In 1882 Pasteur suggested that the causative agent of an infectious disease that was carried by the plant louse, *Phylloxera vitifoliae*, could be used to control phylloxera, which was then plaguing French vineyards. This idea was never successfully applied to this problem, but Pasteur took up this same approach a few years later. In 1860, both Australia and New Zealand had imported the European rabbit. The animals thrived in their new environment, where there were no natural enemies, and soon overran both countries, consuming enormous quantities of grazing plants and posing a serious economic threat to sheep ranchers. In desperation, the government of New South Wales offered a prize of £25,000 for an effective method of controlling the destructive rabbit plague. Pasteur, in competing for this prize, suggested that grass from the area around the rabbit burrows be collected, contaminated with cultures of the chicken cholera bacillus, and spread out in various suitable locations. Pasteur knew that this bacteria (*Pasteurella multocida*) was quite virulent for the European rabbit, and he believed that the ingestion of infected grass would result in clinical disease in the rabbit population.

Shortly after presenting his plan, Pasteur was given the opportunity to test it on a small scale. Madame Pommery, owner of a well-known French champagne firm, complained to Pastuer that his same species of rabbit was becoming increasingly bothersome to winegrowers. Loir, one of Pasteur's trusted laboratory assistants, was sent to the Pommery estate to test the theory. The complete success of this initial effort encouraged Pasteur to send Loir to Australia to test his idea on a larger scale. However, the Australian agriculture department, afraid that the infectious agent would endanger other forms of life, decided not to authorize the tests, and Pasteur's antirabbit offensive was never carried out on a large scale.

Friedrich August Johannes Loeffler (1852–1915) was the first scientist to test Pasteur's approach in the field against a plague of mice. The year was 1892, and the battlefield was Thessaly. This region of north central Greece is one of broad fertile plains, separated from its ancient northern neighbor Macedonia by Mt. Olympus, the traditional home of the gods that rises majestically to a height of almost 10,000 feet. Loeffler described both the land and his adversaries:

> The whole of Thessaly is really one vast plain bordered by mountains, and divided by the range of hills just mentioned into the plain of Larissa and the plain of Trikala. It is traversed from west to east by the river Peneios.... The soil is extremely fertile, heavy, and in many places reddish loam, which is often inundated by the Peneios in winter over a large extent of the country. This vast fertile plain is for the most part the property of large landowners. The population is scanty and the comparatively small number of inhabitants is of course insufficient to cultivate these extenstive flats. Very large districts, perhaps more than two-thirds of the country, lie fallow. The fallow lands are used to pasture large flocks of sheep, goats, and herds of oxen. About every three years the same tracts of land come into cultivation.... In thse extensive fallow fields the voles can multiply undisturbed. Last year the harvest was a good one.... The field voles, which have always been plentiful in Thessaley (the ancient Greeks had their Apollo Smiheus or Myoktonos, the Mouse-destroying God), multiplied because of the good harvest.... By the end of February 1892, they had appeared in larger numbers than for twenty-five years. At the beginning of March 1891, the voles were only beginning to troop from the slopes of the hills and the fallow lands of the cultivated fields. When the sun dried up the fallow fields at the end of May 1891, as happens every year, the mice invaded the cultivated fields and caused such terrible ravages in a short time that last year scarcely any harvest was gathered. The country people were mostly indifferent about the vole-plague. The turkish inhabitants of the country regarded it as a visitation of God, to which one must submit. The notions of the Turks were well illustrated by their sending messengers to Mecca to fetch holy water, with which to sprinkle the fields, and thus, as they supposed, exorcise the mice.

Friedrich Loeffler was born at Frankfort on the Oder, Germany, in 1852. His father, Gottfried Loeffler, was a most distinguished army physician who was a subdirector of the Kaiser Wilhelm academy for military medicine in Berlin, with the military rank of general and the academy rank of professosr. Gottfried Loeffler received the Iron Cross (first class) in recognition of his accomplishments during his military career. After his death, a marble bust testified to his standing at the academy. Friedrich's early education at Marburg and the Royal French College in Berlin was followed by the study of medicine at Würzburg. His studies were interrupted by the Franco-Prussian War, in which he served as a hospital assistant. Loeffler's choice of medicine as a field of study was obviously influenced by his eminent father and by his own inclination to the natural sciences. After the war, Loeffler completed his medical training at the Kaiser Wilhelm academy in Berlin, receiving his medical degree in 1874. The next year he was stationed at Hanover and later at Potsdam, where he practiced medicine while functioning as a sanitary officer. In 1879, shortly after his transfer to the newly established imperial health department in Berlin, he became associated with Robert Koch. His work with Koch, the founder of modern bacteriology in Germany, influenced the entire course of Loeffler's career, an influence Loeffler always appreciated:

> The memory of those days, when we still worked in this room. Koch in the center and we about him, when almost daily new wonders in bacteriology ar ose before our astounded vision, and we, following the brilliant example of our chief, worked from morn to eve and scarcely had regard to our bodily needs—the memory of that time will remain unforgettable to us. Then it was that we learnt what it means to observe and work accurately and with energy to pursue the problem laid before us.

Loeffler's assignment to Berlin placed him at the right place at the right time— at the beginning of the golden era of bacteriology.

Today Loeffler is best remembered for the contributions he made to this golden era during which so many pivotal bacteriological discoveries were made. Loeffler's greatest accomplishment was his work with diphtheria, in which he satisfied Koch's postulates and demonstrated that *Corynebacterium diphtheriae* was responsible for diphtheria.

Although the history of diphtheria dates back to ancient Egypt, the association of a specific bacillus with the false membrane of the pharynx was first made by Klebs in 1883. The following year Loeffler satisfied the three postulates of pathogenesis. First, the organism was identified in its characteristic site in the charaterisitic lesion. Second, the organism was isolated and survived reculturing. Third, inoculation of the pure culture reproduced the disease experimentally. A condensed version of his original report was translated (in the third person) and published by the New Sydenham Society in 1886:

> Loeffler was thus induced to apply the more accurate methods of Koch to the elucidation of the questions as to the significance of the various organisms found in diphtheria, and as to their efficacy in propagating the disease in animals.

In the second class of cases the bacilli first described by Klebs are present. These bacilli occur exclusively over the mucous membrane of the fauces, larynx, and trachea, the mucous membrane being traversed by enormously dilated vessels. Below the masses of bacteria of different kinds which cover the surface, among which may be the streptococcus before referred to, Klebs' bacilli are found arranged in little groups. They become intensely stained with methylene blue.

Material for cultivation was selected from four typical cases in children aged 5, 6, 8 and 9 years, the membrane being taken on the second day of the disease before any treatment had been begun. The false membrane, which was in all cases firmly adherent, was seized with forceps, a portion removed and cut with a freezing microtome. . . . It was from the deeper part that the material was taken for cultivation in all the cases, and that identical organisms were obtained from all patients was proved both by their morphological and their biological characteristics.

Inoculation experiments were made on mice, rats, guinea pigs, rabbits, monkeys, pigeons, hens, and smaller birds, and the behavior of the bacilli towards the various species is a matter of great interest. The modes of infection tried consisted of subcutaneous inoculation, inoculation on the wounded or unharmed mucous membrane and inhalation.

When inoculations were made through the skin or mucous membrane the following results were obtained: rats and mice enjoy complete immunity, while guinea pigs fall easy victims: . . . . Pigeons also are susceptible, and hens behave similarly, but hens and pigeons are not as susceptible as the small birds and cannot be infected through an uninjured mucous membrane. Rabbits do not give such uniform results as the preceding: it would appear from the experiments of Loeffler that death is due in their case to the mechanical effects of the false membrane caused by infection, and that a chemical poison is not developed in the blood, as in the case of guinea pigs.

Loeffler also isolated the causative agent of glanders and once again applied the Koch postulates.

In accordance with Koch's method of cultivation for the bacillus of tubercle, a number of small particles, carefully selected from glanders nodules taken from the lungs and spleen of a horse which had suffered from glanders, were placed, on the 14th of September, in a series of sterilized test tubes containing the blood serum of a horse or sheep. During the first two days no changes were observed on the inoculated surface of the serum. On the third day however, numbers transparent droplets which had formed in places on the surface of the serum were observed in the majority of the test tubes. . . . Similar droplets were found in almost all the test tubes inoculated with glanders material, and always contained the one kind of bacterium. Such being the case, one was naturally induced to test these bacilli as to their causal relation with glanders by inoculation of healthy animals susceptible to the disease. When a successful result was obtained the cultures were further contained through four generations for one month, in order that the objection might not be raised that particles of the original material were present in the vaccinating fluid. On the 14th of October, a small quantity of this fourth cultivation, consisting only of the above described bacilli, was inoculated on the mucous membrane of the nose, and on the two shoulders of an old apparently healthy horse. In forty eight hours the animal began to show signs of high fever. At the inoculated spots deep ulcers developed, from which knotted lymphatic cords extended to the nearest lymphatic glands, so that in about eight days after the inoculation the horse exhibited the pronounced clinical appearance of glanders.

The post mortem was surprising. . . . The fresh glanders material taken from the animal was employed for new cultures. Transparent drops similar to the previous culture developed in three days and contained the above described bacilli. The same bacilli were found after treatment with methylene blue from fresh glanders products taken from the dead horse. During the November the fresh organs from another horse suffering from glanders were examined and the same transparent drop containing bacilli were successfully cultivated from the glanders nodules present in the liver. Again on the 1st of December, in a fourth case, cultures were successfully made from fresh glanders nodules, and the result was in all cases the same.

His other accomplishments included isolation of the bacteria of swine erysipelas and his demonstration that the infectious agent of foot-and-mouth disease passed through filters that retained bacteria, and this led to his introduction of the term *filterable virus.*

In 1888 Loeffler accepted an appointment as professor of hygiene at Greifswald. There he began to study the bacterium of mouse typhoid *(Salmonella typhimurium).* It was this work that eventually led him to travel to Thessaly, where he initiated the first extensive field trials on the use of microbes in the biological control of an animal population.

According to Loeffler, by March 1892 all of the newspapers of Europe carried the story that the plain of Thessaly was besieged by hordes of field mice that threatened the entire harvest. Such episodic visitations were newsworthy, but they were not new. The many accounts of such plagues constitute a chronicle of ineffectual efforts to defeat the countless rodents. As pointed out by Elton, the accounts read much like war reports:

The accounts of these plagues abound in military metaphors, which testify to the serious threat that mice can offer to country people. We read of invasions, advances, attacks on crops, squadrons of mice, campaigns, victories, and defeats. Everything takes place on a huge scale. It is difficult for us in this quiet country [England] to realize that an area of farm-land equal in size to all the plantings made by the British Forestry Commission during the last eighteen years may be ravaged by mice; that the damage runs into millions; that hundreds of villages turn out to make war on the pests; and that this happens, not just once in a generation, but sometimes twice or more in ten years.

As luck would have it, this Thessalian mouse plague coincided with Loeffler's report of his studies on mouse typhoid, in which he suggested that there might well be a new bacteriological method to control field mice. Through its ambassador in Berlin, the Greek government became aware of Loeffler and his work and contacted him, requesting cultures of *S. typhimurium* for use in Thessaly in an attempt to control the field mice. Loeffler immediately realized that this was the perfect chance to give his method of bacteriological control a practical trial.

In his original studies Loeffler had demonstrated that the mouse typhoid bacterium was infectious for both the house mouse and the field mouse but that it was not infectious for other animals, such as cats, rats, rabbits, guinea pigs, swine, small birds, chickens, and pigeons. Loeffler realized that his bacterium would have to be harmless to farm animals if it was to have any value in combating plagues of field mice. His initial studies had shown that fairly large doses of bacteria could be fed to sheep without producing any clinical evidence of desease, and he assumed that animals larger than sheep, such as horses or cows, would also be safe. In fact, he was of the opinion that field trials with *S. typhimurium* could be undertaken with great safety, because sheep were almost the only economically important animals in the besieged area of Thessaly. Loeffler's preliminary studies had also provided other evidence suggesting that the field experiment might well prove successful. This work had shown that mouse typhoid, once established experimentally in mice, would spread among field mice in the field because of further contamination of food sources by the excrement of infected animals. He suggested that the infection could be disseminated even more rapidly and more effectively if the bacilli could be distributed over a wide area in the food of the animals.

This was an opportunity Loeffler did not want to lose. He believed in this idea, and he believed that it was so important that he wanted to carry out the field test himself. So he wrote the Greek ambassador and requested travel funds for himself and for an assistant and a place of residence while conducting the trials. On April 1, 1892, he received word from the Greek government that he was invited to come to Greece, all expenses paid, with an assistant to carry out the trial.

Loeffler left Berlin on April 5, 1892, with his assistant Rudolf Abel. They arrived in Athens 4 days later. There, in the bacteriology laboratories, Dr. Pampoukis showed Loeffler a vole that had been brought from Larissa, the provincial capital of Thessaly. The vole was not of the same species that Loeffler had been working with in Griefswald, but a few inoculation studies showed that the Thessalian vole was even more susceptible than its European counterpart to the bacteria Loeffler had brought with him.

In order to carry out his battle plan, which called for the contamination of food supplies throughout much of Thessaly, Loeffler faced the majot task of producing enormous amounts of virulent bacteria. This proved to be a more formidable problem than he had anticipated. He had hoped to find, somewhere in Athens, a large steam apparatus that could be used to sterilize the large amounts of culture media needed to grow the organism. Unfortunately, this could not be found anywhere in Athens, and Loeffler had to settle for a rather small steam sterilizer located in the kitchen of the university hospital. This small sterilizer presented further problems. The large glass containers he hoped to use could not withstand the heating procedure necessary to effect sterilization, and he was forced to look for a suitable substitute. Finally, Loeffler was forced to use large milk cans, which could withstand the necessary heating, as culture vessels. These worked well, and an amount of *S. typhimurium* sufficient to start the offensive was finally prepared. Loeffler also prepared a number of agar slant cultures of the organism. This was done as a safeguard. If the cultures grown in milk cans spoiled in transit to the fields, he could use such agar cultures to contaminate water and then soak the food in the polluted water.

All of this accomplished, Loeffler, Abel, Pampoukis, and the bacteria arrived in Thessaly on April 18. They were received with mixed emotions by the populace they had come to help. Previous abatement programs, including the use of poisoned food, the distribution of metal traps over the fields, and the application of carbon disulfide, had all proved to be ineffective. The Greek landowners were sophisticated enough to understand Loeffler's plan and were both hopeful and cooperative. The Greek peasants were less sophisticated, less hopeful, and less cooperative. The Turkish landowners believed that the plague was an act of Allah and thus had to be accepted and endured. Because of these problems, the experiments were undertaken on the property of the Greek landowners who were most sympathetic to the design of the program. The apathy of the peasants was in part overcome by eliciting the assistance of the local police force to see to it that the peasants carried out Loeffler's instructions.

In general, Loeffler's plan followed the intended outline. From his headquarters in Larissa, Loeffler and members of his team would travel to one of the estates in the region with large kettles filled with the broth culture previously prepared in Athens. Peasants, sent by the soldiers in the various surrounding towns, brought quantities of bread, which they then soaked in the infected fluid. The infected bread was then carried by the peasants to the selected fields in wicker baskets and distributed around the burrows of voles.

This dispersal procedure was repeated at several different places, and soon reports of large numbers of dead animals were received by the group at Larissa. For Loeffler, such reports constituted adequate evidence that the method worked. Loeffler was satisfied that his approach was proving successful and that it no longer required his personal attention. He left the rest of the program in the hands of his Greek associates and returned to Griefswald.

On May 26 he received a telegram from the president of the vole commission of Larissa that thanked him for the excellent results. IN his own report, Loeffler concluded that *S typhimurium* could be easily, safely, and successfully used to quell plagues of field mice.

Not everyone was so sure that the experiment had been a success. The British committee on voles was much less enthusiastic about the results of this experiment. Two representatives visited Thessaly in January 1893. At the first place they visited, everyone agreed that Loeffler's bacillus was a good poison and was harmless to other animals and to man. But they were equally unanimous in the conclusion that in spite of its application the voles were still as numerous as ever on some parts of the land. In fact, they were informed that on that very morning a steamer was to leave Volo, hired by the Turkish landowners to bring holy water from Mecca with which to sprinkle the infested district. At Larissa itself, the same opinion about the bacillus prevailed, except that Anastassiades, the president of the vole commission, was satisfied that some 7,500 acres of his own land had been cleared of voles.

Pasteur was unconvinced, as his interview with the British committee shows:

> M. Pasteur, while admitting freely the efficacy of the virus in destroying those individual mice which should actually swallow it, had some difficulty in understanding how, in the open country, a sufficient number of these animals could be

made to partake of it so as to make an appreciable impression on the plague. Moreover, without throwing the slightest doubt on Professor Loeffler's skill or accuracy, or on the importance of his discovery of the bacillus of mouse typhus, M. Pasteur pointed out that there was nothing in the reports to prove either the final extirpation of the hordes of voles, or if such had taken place, the connection between the employment of the virus and the disappearance of the voles. It was usual, he said, for these outbreaks to diminish either from natural causes or from some epixootic disease, as suddenly as they arose; and it had not been established that Professor Loeffler's operations had done more than synchronize with the abatement of the plague.

Loeffler never publicly replied to these criticisms and never again returned to the field mouse abatement. In 1893, another strain of *Salmonella*, the so-called Danysz virus, which was considered to be more effective than *S. typhimurium*, was found.

Extensive field trials with the new *Salmonella* were begun in France, and from that time until the present there have been numerous commercial products containing various species of *Salmonella* that have been recommended for rodent-abatement programs. Unfortunately, there has never been unanimity of opinion on the efficacy of any of these products. Often they have been employed to a saturation point, much as a chemical poison would be used. Under these circumstances they unquestionably kill enormous numbers of mice, but they do not accomplish the original goal of biological control: induction of a large-scale epidemic from a point source.

The gradual realization that the *Salmonella* employed have been far from innocuous for man has argued against their use in biological control programs, and products containing these microorganisms have been largely abandoned.

Following his return to Griefswald, Loeffler continued his basic bacteriological studies. From 1903 to 1907 he was rector of the university, and then he returned to Berlin as director of the Robert Koch Institute of Infectious Diseases. With the outbreak of World War I, he returned to military service as a consultant to the military hospitals, with the rank of surgeon general, but he died a few months later.

The most famous attempt to control an animal population with an infectious disease concerned the same rabbit problem that had originally attracted Pasteur. The disease used to kill the rabbits was not that suggested by Pasteur, but myxomatosis. Myxomatosis gets its name from the slimy tumors, myxomas, that typify the disease. It is a viral disease, and a most peculiar one. The virus is dangerous to only one species in the entire animal kingdom, but for that species it is nearly 100% fatal. The susceptible species, of course, is the common European rabbit, the well-known backyard pet and the principal game animal of France. It is a source of meat, furs, and experimental subjects in biological laboratories throughout the world.

The disease was first discovered in Uruguay in 1896 by the Italian bacteriologist G. Sanarelli, whose laboratory rabbits at the hygiene institute in Montevideo were dying of a strange new disorder. Sanarelli described the disease, named it infectious myxomatosis, and guessed correctly that it was caused by a virus.

In 1942–43, H. de Beaurepaïre Aragao of the Oswaldo Cruz Institute in Rio de Janeiro established two critical facts about the natural history of myxomatosis. He showed that the native *Sylvilagus* rabbit of Brazil harbored the virus and that mosquitoes could transmit the infection from these rabbits to European rabbits who were susceptible to it.

The effects of the infection in European rabbits have been studied by intradermal inoculation of rabbits with a standard dose that it believed to approximate the natural method of infection by a mosquito bite. Three or 4 days after the inoculation, a small, red, hard spot appears at the site of the injection, and the spot slowly increases in size. On the fifth day the rabbit's eyelids begin to swell, and soon its eyes are swollen shut as the rabbit's entire face becomes severely swollen. Swelling then appears in the anogenital region, and the animal survives long enough, the typical gelatinous tumors begin to appear all over the surface of its body. Usually, however, the animal dies before this stage is reached. The rabbit becomes lethargic, then stuporous; its respiration and pulse rate slow down, and death commonly occurs on the ninth or tenth day.

Two things made the myxoma virus an ideal instrument for controlling the rabbit nuisance in Australia. In the first place, this virus apparently does not harm any other animal. In the second place, the disease is amazingly lethal to the European rabbit. One investigator has said that every last rabbit of 2,000 he had infected in the laboratory died of the disease, and others have reported that only two or three of the hundreds exposed in their experiments have recovered.

The first suggestion that the myxoma virus might be of value in combating the Australian plague of European rabbits was made by the Brazilian investigator Aragao in 1918. The Australian authorities, who had vetoed Pasteur's suggestion that chicken cholera bacteria be used, were interested. Their concerns about the safety of other animals that had led them to reject Pasteur's scheme had to be answered for this agent. As a result, they deferred any extensive testing of the idea until it was known that the virus could not be harmful to others animals. These experiments were carried out between 1933 and 1937, and they confirmed that myxomatosis infected only rabbits.

In 1950, field trials were carried out at three different sites in the well-watered region of Australia's Murray Valley. These experiments, like some earlier ones carried out in similar areas of south Australia in 1937, seemed to end in failure. At the end of the trials the rabbit population was much larger than it had been at the beginning, despite the fact that numerous animals had died of myxomatosis. The Australian authorities were virtually convinced that this attempt at rabbit abatement had been a failure and that myxomatosis would not spread well enough in the field to prove useful in such programs.

Five days after the study was completed, reports began to trickle in that sick rabbits with swollen heads were being seen in the areas near the test sites. Soon the trickle became a flood, so that when the first summer's outbreak was over, infected rabbits had been found over an area totaling 500,000 square miles. The next summer, another widespread epidemic occurred. By the summer of 1952–53, the disease had spread to every part of southeastern Australia in which there were enough rabbits to support an epizootic. It is estimated that within 3 years the 500 million rabbits that had been plaguing this part of Australia had been reduced to 10% to 15% of their original numbers.

In 1952, French microbiologists, encouraged by these results, returned to the Pommery estate, where Pasteur had tried to curb the rabbits with a bacteria. This time they used myxoma virus. Unfortunately, this time the microbial parasite failed to stay within the estate on which it was liberated. In the winter of 1952–53, myxomatosis broke out in a number of areas in France, and then the disease spread over the country, with much the same rapidity and destructiveness it had shown in southeastern Australia. The disease and disease-carrying rabbits and mosquitoes do not respect national boundaries any more than they abide by estate boundaries. Soon, cases of myxomatosis were reported in game rabbits in Holland, Belgium, Germany, and even England.

All this while the plagues of mice have continued to come and go. For unknown reasons, the voles or lemmings still suddenly increase in numbers and then, after a year or two, having destroyed crops and human hopes and aspirations, they disappear. But they will return. They always have.

NOTES

Loeffler's own report on his campaign in Thessaly against the voles was published in German. English translations of parts of this can be found in C. Elton's *Voles, Mice and Lemmings* (Oxford: Clarendon Press, 1942). This unassuming book is the best single source in any language on plagues of mice. The most thorough review of Loeffler's mouse episode is D. H. Howard's "Friedrich Loeffler and the Thessalian Field Mouse Plagues of 1892" (*Journal of the History of Medicine* 32:272–281, 1963). The most readable description of the use of myxomatosis against rabbits is F. Fenner's *The Rabbit Plague (Scientific American* 90:30–35, 1954).

Vaginismus and Other Medical Satires

False delicacy must not be allowed for one moment to prevent us looking this condition straight in the face.

F. H. Champneys, "Notes of a Clinical Lecture on Vaginismus"
Clinical Journal (1:42–44, 1892–93)

There's a sucker born every minute.

Usually attributed to P. T. Barnum but reputedly first said by Chicago gambler Mike McDonald.

Vaginismus and Other Medical Satires

Vaginismus

Through the courtesy of the Editor of The Canadian Medical and Surgical Journal, we are in receipt of the following note:

Dear Sir:

The reading of an admirably written and instructive editorial in the Philadelphia Medical News for 24th November, on forms of vaginismus, has reminded me of a case in point which bears out, in an extraordinary way, the statements therein contained. When in practice at Pentonville, Eng., I was sent for about 11 p.m., by a gentleman whom, on my arriving at his house, I found in a state of great perturbation, and the story he told me was briefly as follows:

At bedtime, when going to the back kitchen to see if the house was shut up, a noise in the coachman's room attracted his attention, and, going in, he discovered to his horror that the man was in bed with one of the maids. She screamed, he struggled, and they rolled out of bed together and made frantic efforts to get apart, without success. He was a big, burly man, over six feet, and she was a small woman weighing not more than ninety pounds. She was moaning and screaming, and seemed in great agony, so that, after several fruitless attempts to get them apart, he sent for me. When I arrived I found the man standing up and supporting the woman in his arms, and was quite evident that his penis was tightly locked in her vagina, and any attempt to dislodge it was accompanied by much pain on the part of both. It was, indeed, a case "De cohesione in coitu." I applied water, and then ice, but ineffectually, and at last sent for chloroform, a few whiffs of which sent the woman to sleep, relaxed the spasm, and relieved the captive penis, which was swollen, livid, and in a state of semi-erection, which did not go down for several hours, and for days the organ was extremely sore. The woman recovered rapidly, and seemed none the worse.

I am sorry that I did not examine if the sphincter ani was contracted, but I did not think of it. In this case there must have been also spasm of the muscle at the orifice, as well as higher up; for the penis seemed nipped low down, and this contraction, I think, kept the blood retained and the organ erect. As an instance of Jago's "beast with two backs," the picture was perfect. I have often wondered how it was, considering with what agility the man can, under certain circumstances, jump up that Phineas, the son of Eleazar, was able to thrust his javelin through the man and the Midianitish woman; (vide Exodus); but the occurrence of such cases as the above may offer a possible explanation.

Yours truly,

Egerton Y. Davis
Ex. U.S. Army

Caughnawaga, Quebec, 4th December, 1884.

This letter appeared in an issue of *Medical News* in 1884. *Medical News* was then a most prestigious journal. It was the oldest American medical journal, having been founded in 1827, and there were only two older English-language journals: *The*

Edinburgh Medical Journal and *The Lancet*. This letter had been stimulated by an editorial that had appeared in *Medical News* a few weeks earlier:

AN UNCOMMON FORM OF VAGINISMUS.

The word cunnus, signifying the female pudendum, was said to have been used by "the more lascivious poets," and was condemned by Cicero, in one of his orations, as an obscene word. Though Horace does not deserve to be placed in this class, yet he made use of the word: *Fuit ante Helenum cunnus teterrima belli causa*. Nevertheless, it has a classic derivation, probably coming from *kveiv*—to be pregnant—and for many years had a place in anatomy; indeed, up to the present some writers speak of the constrictor cunni muscle, but most now designate the muscular structure which contracts the vaginal entrance as the bulbo-cavernosi muscles; these are the vaginal sphincter.

The late Dr. Sims, in a paper communicated to the London Obstetrical Society by Dr. Tyler Smith in 1861, stated that, by the term vaginismus, he proposed to designate "an involuntary, spasmodic closure of the mouth of the vagina, attended by such excessive supersensitiveness as to form a complete barrier to coition." Dr. Sims did not describe a new disease—indeed, he disclaimed any such attempt. Dr. Louis Debrand, who has recently published an important monograph, *Des Retre-cissements du Conduit Vulvo-Vaginal*, states that Huguier, in 1834, was the first to describe spasmodic contraction of the vaginal sphincter. Nevertheless, though Dr. Sims only recalled attention to a disorder which others had observed, he gave it a name so suitable that it at once received general acceptance, and is sure to keep its place in medical nomenclature.

But while the name was received with such favor, its definition as given by Dr. Sims was soon found to be too narrow. For example, in a case of vaginismus recently under our observation (the subject had been married several months, and coition had been impossible) there was very great suffering, especially marked at the monthly periods, in the anal sphincter, violent cramp of this muscle, accompanied with painful defecation, although there was no local disease to be discovered here, and the affection was cured by the treatment of the vaginismus, using this word as previous defined.

Hildebrandt, who has written, in Billroth's *Handbuch der Frauenkrankheiten*, probably the best article upon vaginismus to be found, remarks: "Most frequently the constrictor cunni is the seat of this cramp. From the anatomical position of this muscle the necessarily following results are the impossibility of coitus, the application of a speculum, even the introduction of the exploring finger." He then adds that, in the further progress of the disease, there occurs cramp of the anal sphincter, in which the patient has a sensation of swelling, rigid enlargement, tension, spasmodic jerking, and difficult and painful defecation. He describes this spasm as extending to other muscles, or to groups of muscles, forming the pelvic floor; in rare cases all the muscles are affected. He states that cramp of the levator ani may cause contraction of the upper part of the vagina, so that a speculum, or a swollen glans penis, as in coition, may be forcibly retained.

The form of vaginismus last mentioned has recently been considered again by Henrichsen in the *Archive für Gynäkologie*. The author refers to the observations of Scanzoni, and those of Hildebrandt, in which the penis was retained captive by a woman's genital organs, after coitus, by a phenomenon analogous to that observed in certain animals especially the dog. He states that while Scanzoni thought this phenomenon due to the constrictor of the vagina, Hildebrandt attributes it to the levator ani, for the constrictor of the vagina would oppose the intromission of the penis, and it is not at all probable that spasm of the latter muscle could retain the member already introduced, especially a part of it which is smaller than the glans.

Debrand, *op. cit.*, quotes from Revillout a case in which the contraction was about two inches from the vaginal entrance, and a little below the neck of the uterus and the vaginal cul-de-sacs; there seemed to be two muscular bands at this point, one on each side, which contracting, narrowed the canal; the contraction was voluntary.

It is somewhat remarkable that in the recent study of vaginismus affecting the canal in its middle or upper portion, spasmodic elytrostenia, as it is called by Debrand, no reference is made to the facts that it was observed many years ago, and that the very comparison as to the captive human penis now made was then used. Schurigius, in 1729, wrote *De cohaesione in coitu*, and referred to it as analogous to the retention of the penis noticed in animals; he quotes Lannius as stating it to be a spasmodic affection of the female genitals. Riolanus describes it as a grasping of the penis by the mouth of the womb after menstruation, "and retaining it, as is done in dogs." Diemerbroc, in 1687, also mentioned the disease.

It is well for us to be grateful for all additions to medical knowledge, but it is also well for us not to neglect the observations of past ages, and to remember that rediscoveries are probably more frequent than discoveries.

This editorial, which preceded a report on an address given before the New York Medical Association by the renowned Austin Flint, was written by a well-respected Philadelphia professor of obstetrics, Dr. Theophilus Parvin. The reply was written by the man destined to become the most dominant and most respected physician and teacher of his generation, William Osler, who was later to become Sir William Osler. Osler, it seems, found Parvin's editorial to border on the absurd. As such, it required an absurd reply, and Osler was just the man to produce such a reply, but not over his own name. For such adventures, Osler reserved the pseudonym "Egerton Yorrick Davis, Late U.S. Army Surgeon," a title most reminiscent of "John H. Watson, M.D., Late of Her Majesty's Army."

While this and other E.Y. Davis diversions are almost invariably omitted in serious discussions of Osler's life, this letter is at other times presented as one of the most successful of all medical hoaxes. But was it really a hoax? A hoax is usually considered to be a humorous or mischievous deception, a trick most often in the form of a fabricated story played on someone for sport, a sort of literate practical joke. A hoax, to truly be a hoax, must have no element of fraud in it. A fraud, in this sense, is a form of deceit or deception deliberately carried out in order to gain some advantage, usually monetary, in a dishonest manner. The difference between a hoax and a fraud is not in the content of the deception but in its intent. A true hoax is carried out solely for amusement, and the only cost to its target is embarrassment. A fraud is designed to cost the victim more than just his response to its mischief. Certainly this letter made no attempt to defraud Parvin, who had not even signed the editorial, and in that sense it does qualify as a hoax, not a fraud. But was its intention deception or satire? Osler's, or Davis's case has often been quoted in serious gynecologic journals and textbooks as a documented instance of vaginismus associated with "De cohesione in coitu." The fact that many so-called experts over the generations have been taken in by this brief case report does not prove that it was originally designed to deceive the reader, that it was truly meant to be a hoax from its inception.

Rather than a hoax, "Vaginismus" was a satire. A satire is a literary composition meant to expose or ridicule someone else's follies or abuses. If the entire conception of the satire is subtle enough, its targets may believe it. Any hoax that results is due to the foibles of the audience, not to the intent of the author. This can best be seen in a more recent medical satire that unaccountably actually deceived at least one prominent medical author.

In 1957, a brief biography of Emile Coudé, signed merely R.P., appeared in *The Leech*, a hard-to-obtain journal of limited circulation published by the students of the Welsh national school of medicine at Cardiff, Wales. This article appeared as the first biography in a series: "Lesser Known Names in Medicine and Surgery."

EMILE COUDÉ (1800–1870)

Although the catheter he designed is in common use today, little is known of Coudé in this country.

He was born the son of a country doctor in the small town of Villeneuve-la-Comtesse, near the west coast port of La Rochelle. As a boy he loved to play around the ancient castle with its fourteenth century keep, which is still a well-known tourist attraction of the region.

As he grew up he attended lessons in the local school, but in his spare time he loved to accompany his father on his rounds in the small coach-and-pair. Occasionally he would be allowed inside a house to look at a patient with his father (a special treat, this), but usually he had to wait outside, looking after the horses.

On one of these occasions, Pierre, the larger of the two horses, was stung by a wasp. Frightened, he bolted, causing the other horse, Phillippe, to run off as well. Emile was in the carriage at the time. He tried in vain to halt the horses by pulling on the reins, until, as a wheel went into a small pot-hole in the rough country road, he was thrown off. He was not badly hurt, but a long gash on his right leg left him a scar there for the rest of his days.

As time went by, Emile spent more and more time with his father, visiting patients. In his twenties, he went to Paris to study under the great Dupuytren at Hotel Dieu. Like most people he found Dupuytren's nature unattractive, though he was certainly a great surgeon and teacher. Coudé himself was one of the "brigand's" assistants at the first removal of a mandible ever performed. It is not known exactly how long Coudé spent in Paris. He said later that although he had undoubtedly learned much from Dupuytren, he had learned much more from his father.

On his return to his native town, Emile Coudé played an ever-increasing part in his father's practice. But he had always been interested in surgery, and so in 1832 he accepted the post of assistant surgeon at Niort, seventeen miles north of his home town. It was here that he designed the catheter which bears his name.

In cases of retention of urine he found the catheters then available were difficult to use, being either perfectly straight and rigid, or else, as he put it in his memoirs, "bent to many weird shapes, as if a catheter should copy exactly the bends of the male urethra."

After trying many different designs, he hit upon the well-known "bicoude" catheter. Other doctors referred to it as the "Coude" catheter, but its inventor's natural modesty caused him to add the prefix "bi" (because it had two bends) in order to hide his name. The first published description of the instrument appeared in 1835.

Coudé had married in 1830, and his son Robert began to learn medicine from his father, as Emile had done before him. When Emile Coudé retired in 1865, his son was already an assistant surgeon at Bordeaux. Before he died, in 1870, Emile expressed a wish to be buried in the place of his birth. He was buried on June the fourteenth and his tombstone can still be seen in the small cemetery attached to the beautiful thirteenth century church at Villeneuve-la-Comtesse.

This article in the student journal was complete with footnotes and was documented by the only surviving portrait of Emile Coudé (Fig. 1), obviously taken at the height of his career and reprinted with permission of "Laraboussie et Cie" of Bordeaux, the publishers of Coudé's alleged 1868 autobiography, "*Ma Vie et Mon Travail.*"

It is difficult to conceive that anyone would be taken in by this satire on medical biographies and the use of eponyms that have little significance for today's physicians. The coudé (not Coudé) catheter is a slightly bent catheter that is shaped that way to allow easier passage through the male urethra. The name of this bent instrument comes from the French word for bent, *coudé*. It was a satire pure and

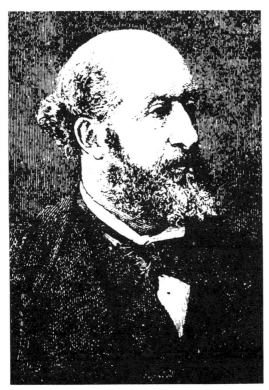

FIG. 1. The only known portrait of Emile Coudé. (Courtesy of Dr. R. Pash and the editor of *The Leech*.)

simple, published in a student journal filled with other lampoons of the medical establishment, with no intention to deceive. But Barnum was absolutely right. No less an authority than the late Hamilton Bailey was taken in, as the following letter to the *British Medical Journal* (I:513, 1958) attests:

COUDE CATHETER

Sir—In volume 6 of the winter number of the Leech—the journal of the Cardiff Medical Students' Club—there appeared an article on Emile Coudé. 1800–70, a surgeon of Niort, France, who it was alleged, invented, and in 1835 published an account of the coudé catheter. This biography was written in a serious and restrained vein, and was replete with two references, one to the autobiography of Emile Coudé, and another to *Le Mois Medical* for a description of the invention. In addition, the article contained a reproduction of a woodcut purporting to be a likeness of the inventor.

We have been able to prove that the whole of this article is a fabrication, and the references are fictitious. To expose this deception is of practical importance. As a result of the hoax, a number of pages of the 11th edition of *A Short Practice of Surgery* that were passed for press have had to be reset in as far as the capital "C" of Coudé is concerned, and biographical footnotes to Emile Coudé deleted.

To save others from falling into this mire, we hope that you will publish this letter. The coude catheter was invented by Louis Mercier, 1811–82, the eminent Paris urologist, so well known for his description of the interureteric bar. Mercier announced the invention of the coude catheter in 1836 and of the bi-coude catheter in 1841. Being translated, coude (the adjective) means bent: coude (the noun) means elbow.—We are, etc.

> Hamilton Bailey,
> W.J. Bishop, Editor Medical History
> A. Clifford Morson,
> President, Société Internationale
> d'Urologie

In a subsequent reply to this angry note, Peter Birkett, a former editor of *The Leech*, pointed out that any familiarity with the source would have made the satirical intent of the article on Coudé obvious. The subjects of the biographical sketches that had appeared in *The Leech* had included Johannes Haemolyticus, or Giovanni Emolitico (1678–1726), and Staphylococcus of Alexandria (c. 273–200 B.C.), whose names were said to be enshrined in *Streptococcus haemolyticus pyogenes* and *Staphylococcus aureus*. Birkett closed his letter with the hope these other biographies did not lead to similar confusion among historians of bacteriology. Birkett, of course, was right. As far as I know, no textbook of bacteriology has ever made reference to either Johannes Haemolyticus or Staphylococcus.

It seems that Hamilton Bailey had no one to blame but himself for having allowed such an obvious satirical fabrication to deceive him. At the cost of some public embarrassment to himself, and also at the cost of some increased expenditures by his publisher, the matter of the coudé catheter finally appears to have been straightened out. But has it been? The following appeared in *The Lancet* (2:456, 1958) shortly after Bailey's angry missive:

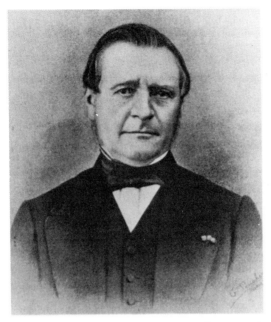

FIG. 2. Photograph of Louis Auguste Mercier (1811–1882). (Courtesy of L. J. T. Murphy, *The History of Urology.* Springfield, Ill.: Charles C Thomas, 1972.)

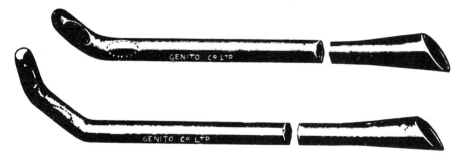

FIG. 3. Mercier's original coudé and bicoudé catheters. (Courtesy of Genito-Urinary Manufacturing Co., Ltd., London.)

Sir—I am a French surgeon who makes his holiday in your so beautiful country and I borrow the pen of my landlady to write to you very quick because I see in your journal a letter which makes me very sad. I think the three gentlemens which write this letter essay to kill in one foul swoop, as you say in your language, so expressive, the sacret memory of the Illustrious Emile Coudé, of who I have the honour to be his grand nephew. It is only last week ago when my assistant at the Salpetriere say to me that there is a patient who cannot pass the water in the antechamber. "The catheter" I cry. "Alas" responds he "I have already try" showing me the straight catheter of M. Jacques. "Imbecile! give me the catheter of my Uncle Coude"—at last! the water she come and again a little more of glory is added to a name which the Société Internationale d'Urologie should revere but would make to fall into the mire. "Over my dead corpse" I cry and sign myself.

Hercule Coudé

Coudé Rebent,
Blackspool-sur-mer

The editors felt that some further reply was needed:

"They fool me to the top of my bent." Thus, with Hamlet, must be thinking the ghost of the illustrious Emile Coudé. His grandnephew, M. Hercule Coudé, has done us service in keeping his name to the fore; but, alas, he falls into the popular error of attributing the straight catheter to M. Jacques.

It is natural to associate catheters with the French, but in this case the catheter is English. Its date of origin is unknown, but it was widely used in the 18th century when, for obvious reasons, it was known simply as "the jakes." In the Victorian era feelings against the name ran high, and it was impossible to move in urological circles without becoming involved in heated arguments. The climax was reached at a certain meeting when it was decided to consign the jakes to oblivion. This so affected a French visitor that he leapt to his feet with the now famous ejaculation: "Eurethra!" Called to the rostrum, this man, M. Jacques, gave an impassioned speech in which he emplored the audience to consider the patient before any matter of prudery. He saved the day and since then the spelling of the catheter has been "Jacques."

The most famous satire that became accepted as a hoax was created by the fertile mind of H.L. Mencken in 1917. In one of his daily syndicated columns, Mencken invented a playful, satirical history of the bathtub in America. According to Mencken, the first bathtub in America with hot and cold running water was installed in the home of Adam Thompson, a grain merchant in Cincinnati, on December 20, 1842. Millard Fillmore was then vice president under Zachary Taylor and allegedly visited Cincinnati during a political stumping sojourn and was a guest in the house of Adam Thompson. While staying there, Fillmore, who was later to become the most obscure of all U.S. presidents, risked a plunge in the Thompson tub. Because he experienced no ill effects from his daring venture and actually enjoyed his dip, Fillmore "became an ardent advocate of the new invention, and, on succeeding to the presidency . . . instructed his secretary of war, Gen. Charles M. Conrad, to invite tenders for the construction of a bathtub in the White House." Mencken had called his article "A Neglected Anniversary" and claimed that he had written it because no one else had done anything to call attention to the 75th anniversary of the installation of America's first bathtub in Cincinnati on December 20, 1842. It was not this aspect of the satire that appealed to Mencken's readers. People across the nation were attracted by Mencken's claim that Fillmore had installed the first White House bathtub and had helped popularize bathing in America. This was pictured as a heroic event, because most doctors were reported to have been outspokenly opposed to bathtubs, fearing that they might be injurious to health. Most other politicians were pictured as opposing a bathtub in the White House as undemocratic.

Mencken's story was widely read, and the little-known Fillmore became known as our first clean president. The fact that California had been admitted to the union during his term in office was overshadowed by his accomplishment in having installed that first White House bathtub. Many people were deceived and continued to be deceived by this satire, accepting it as truth, including even Hans Zinsser in his 1935 classic *Rats, Lice and History*. All this occurred despite the fact that in 1926 Mencken published another column in which he insisted that "A Neglected Anniversary" had been nothing more than a spoof: "If there are any facts in it, they got there accidentally and against my design." Should Mencken be blamed for Zinsser's error? Of course not.

P. J. Wingate, in his "H. L. Mencken's Unneglected Anniversary," has set the record straight on White House bathtubs. The first one was installed during the presidency of Andrew Jackson. Despite a variety of both scholarly and popular corrections of the facts, the Fillmore myth goes on. In an article printed January 7, 1977, Fillmore's birthday, the *Philadelphia Inquirer* called Fillmore "a statesman, scholar, patriot and the finest plumber who ever lived in the White House." Fillmore, in fact, was a statesman, a scholar, and a patriot of considerable distinction. In his one term as president during the turbulent early 1850s, when controversy over slavery threatened to destroy the nation, he served the country most admirably. His talent in conciliation helped bring California into the union.

The assertion that Fillmore was a scholar is also soundly based, despite the fact that he neither attended college nor graduated from high school. In a manner reminiscent of Abraham Lincoln, he educated himself by a rigorous program of home study. Again, like his more famous successor, he was a successful lawyer. After leaving the presidency, he served for many years as chancellor of the University of Buffalo. Despite these accomplishments, he once declined an honorary degree from Oxford University because the degree would have been written in Latin: "I had not the advantage of classical education," he wrote a friend, "and no man should accept a degree he cannot read." However, he was never a plumber.

If satirical articles sometime merge into hoax, deception, and even fraud, in other instances serious contributions to the medical literature have been treated as satire. In *Chest* (67:215–216, 1975), Caroline and Schwartz published a case report entitled "Chicken Soup, Rebound and Relapse of Pneumonia." In it they presented the history of a 47-year-old previously healthy male physician who presented with right-middle-lobe pneumonia that initially improved on a regimen of chicken soup, 500 ml p.o. every 4 hours. Like all physicians, as soon as he felt better he discontinued his medication instead of finishing the prescribed course. Soon he was admitted to a hospital with severe bilateral pneumonia that was refractory to medical treatment and eventually required thoracotomy. These authors reviewed the history of chicken soup as a medicinal agent. The therapeutic efficacy of chicken soup was discovered several thousand years ago when an epidemic that was fatal to firstborn Egyptian males entirely spared an ethnic minority residing in the same area. Epidemiologic studies carried out at the time revealed that one of the most significant ($p < 0.0001$) differences between the Egyptians and the other group (later to be known as Hebrews) was that the diet of the group not afflicted by the epidemic contained large amounts of a preparation made by boiling chicken with vegetables and herbs.

Over the centuries, the efficacy of chicken soup has been unquestioned by its users. Whereas the dietary laws given to Moses at Mount Sinai placed restrictions on 19 different types of fowl, no such restrictions were placed on chicken. Although it had been claimed by Dr. Caroline's grandmother that the recipe for chicken soup was transmitted to Moses on the same occasion, but later was relegated to the oral tradition when the Scriptures were canonized, this hypothesis is not well substantiated. After tracing its use through the ages and its manufacture, "largely in the hands of private individuals, and standardization has proved nearly impossible," these authors turned to its pharmacology:

> readily absorbed after oral administration, achieving peak serum levels in two hours and persisting in detectable levels for up to 24 hours. Parenteral administration is not recommended. The metabolic fate of the agent is not well understood, although varying proportions are excreted by the kidneys, and dosage should be appropriately adjusted in patients with renal failure. Chicken soup is distributed widely throughout body tissues and breakdown products having antimicrobial efficacy cross the blood brain barrier.

Its side effects are "minimal, consisting primarily of mild euphoria which rapidly remits on discontinuation of the agent." Caroline and Schwartz concluded that the relapse had been due to inadequacy of the original course of therapy, and they suggested that a full 10-day course be used in the future. A serious (nearly fatal, in fact) case history such as this is no more a satire than R. P.'s Coudé biography was a hoax, or even E. Y. Davis's "Vaginismus."

Egerton Yorrick Davis was Osler's nom de plume, which he invented for jest and used for satire. Like Coudé, Davis has taken on an existence of his own. Osler is at least partly to blame for this. In a handwritten note, Osler gave some biographical data:

> I never could understand about Egerton Yorrick Davis. He is represented to have practised at Caughnawaga nearly opposite Montreal, where his collections were stored in the Guildhall. Some have said that he was a drunken old reprobate, but the only occasion on which I met him, he seemed a peaceable enough old rascal. One thing is certain, he was drowned in the Lachine Rapids in 1884, and the body was never recovered. He had a varied life—in the U.S. Army; in the North West; among the Indians; as a general practitioner in the north of London. I knew his son well—a nice mild-mannered fellow, devoted to his father. . . .
>
> I heard nothing more from Davis until I went to Philadelphia. I was on the staff of the Medical News, and Parvin in 1884 and 1885 was very interested in the action of the perinaeal muscles. One day I met Minis Hays the Editor, who said; "By the way, do you know Egerton Y. Davis who lives somewhere near Montreal? Parvin is delighted as he has sent the report of a case just such as he thought possible." I said, "Hays, for Heaven's sake! Don't print anything from that man Davis: I know he is not a reputable character. Ross and Roddick know him well." "Too late now," Hays said, "the journal is printed off." So the letter appeared. The case has gone into literature and is often quoted. . . .
>
> Some went so far as to say that I was Davis, and the rumour got about in Philadelphia. I never but once met the man. Afterwards I often used his name when I did not wish to be known. I would sign my name in the Hotel Registers as "E. Y. Davis, Caughnawaga." Once at Atlantic City after I had had broncho-

pneumonia I registered under that name immediately after Mrs. Osler and Revere. I had been there a week when a man came up and said: "Are you Dr. Osler? I have been looking for you for a week: your secretary said you were away and not to be got at. My son is ill here and I wished you to see him." He said to Cadwallader Biddle, "Who is that fellow Davis all the time with Mrs. Osler?"—and was furious when he found that I had registered under that name. They tell in Montreal many jokes about Davis, and father many of them on me. I am always sorry that I did not see more of him, and that I never visited his collections at the Guildhall, Caughnawaga.

In 1949, during the Osler centennial celebration, a letter from Davis's granddaughter Marlene Yorrick Davis surfaced. Like Emile Coudé's grandnephew Hercule, Marlene tried to straighten out the record:

The Guildhall,
Caughnawaga
Quebec, Canada
24th May, 1949.

My dear Sir:
    I am writing this in the Guildhall in the peace that comes over me when I am in the company of my grandfather's mind, if not of his body—surrounded by the famous Egerton Yorrick Davis collection. As I look at some of its treasures, the skull of Plato and the lower jaw of Julius Caesar with its beautiful gold bridgework, the bottle of the waters of Lethe, a chip off Charon's Oar, Aesculapius's thermometer, as well as Dr. Harvey's blood pressure apparatus, and the thesis of Dr. Radcliffe of Oxford on pneumococcal pneumonia (that they gave him the gold-head cane for),—my eyes fill with tears as I think how hard grandpa had to work to get them. How Sir William Osler loved him, and how they used to linger over these old things. Dr. Osler said, I know, that he only met him once, and referred to him in a curious way, "old rogue," I think he called him, but of course we in the family understood that they went off on secret sprees together, like the one in Atlantic City that I think Dr. Cushing must have written about in his book.
    My father was a steady-going man, a doctor too like his dad. He always used to say that it was the bad example that his father Egerton and that man Dr. Osler set him that made him keep to the narrow path.
    Seeing something in the papers about Sir William Osler's being born one or two hundred years ago made me write. I'm looking at grandfather's portrait that hangs in this beautiful room—him, surrounded by the Indians that he treated so kindly. So I send my respects, because I know grand-dad would have wanted it.
                                        Yours Truly,

(signed)   Marlene Yorrick Davis

Marlene, like all other descendants, retained the old family name Yorrick, which could be traced back to Elizabethan times and was mentioned in *Hamlet*: "Alas, poor Yorrick! I knew him, Horatio: a fellow of infinite jest, of most excellent fancy."

E. Y. Davis authored more than one satirical commentary in *Medical News*. In 1886 an editorial was published signed E. Y. D. that discussed the transfer of an extrauterine pregnancy into an intrauterine pregnancy by external application of electricity. This was brought about by several reports of such occurrences published by well-known obstetricians. In this short editorial Osler demonstrated a more accurate knowledge of the physiology and endocrinology of pregnancy than the practicing obstetricians. He knew that the uterus enlarged as much when the fetus was extrauterine as it ordinarily did in the early months of a normal intrauterine pregnancy.

Osler always believed that he was the major victim of the E. Y. Davis affair, because it made editors suspicious of his obstetrical interests, especially in regard to the infamous "baby on the track."

In 1886, while he was vacationing in northwestern Canada, Osler heard about the abrupt birth of a child in the WC of a railroad train while the train was in motion. Osler, according to his own words, learned of the delivery just 2 days after the fact while on the same train. At his request the conductor stopped the train at the station to which the mother had been taken immediately after the event. As luck would have it, both mother and child were still in the region. Dr. Osler interviewed the mother, inspected the bruises on the baby, who, all things considered, seemed no worse from the experience, and obtained affidavits from the conductor and several others who had witnessed the affair firsthand. After completing his vacation, Osler wrote up the tale and sent it to Gould, editor of *Anomalies and Curiosities of Medicine*, with the assurance that he not only could vouch for its truth but also had affidavits to prove it. Gould, like many of Osler's contemporaries, knew of E. Y. D. and Osler's fondness for practical jokes. He was hesitant to accept the report at face value, and he suggested to Osler that the child was born not in the water closet of the train but in the brain of W. O. with E. Y. Davis as midwife. He did agree to publish the account if Osler would send the affidavits. Because Dr. Osler was unable to find the illusive affidavits, all that Gould published was this statement: "There was recently a rumor, probably a newspaper fabrication, that a woman while at stool in a railway car gave birth to a child which was found alive on the track afterward." However, a full report was published in the *Canada Medical and Surgical Journal* and later was abstracted in the *Medical Record* and *New York Medical Journal*. The full report, published in 1888 under the name of William Osler, was as follows:

> an interesting experience which I had in the Northwest in 1886, which is worth placing on record. Mr. Fred Brydges had kindly met our party at the Portage to take us over the Manitoba and North Western Road, and he mentioned two days before, a woman, while in the water closet on the train, had given birth to a child which had dropped to the track and had been found alive some time after. I was so incredulous that he ordered the conductor to stop the train at the station to which the woman had been taken that I might see her and corroborate the story. I found mother and child in the care of the stationmaster's wife, and obtained the following history:
>
> She was aged about 28, well developed, of medium size, and had had two previous labours which were not difficult. She had expected her confinement in a week or ten days, and had got on the train to go to see her husband, who was

working down the track. Having a slight diarrhea she went to the water-closet, and while on the seat, labour pains came on and the child dropped from her. Hearing a noise and groaning, the conductor forced open the door and found the woman on the floor in an exhausted condition, with just strength enough to tell him that the baby was somewhere on the track, and to ask him to stop the train, which was running at the rate of about 20 miles an hour. The baby was found alive off the side of the track a mile or more away, and with the mother was left at the station where I saw her. She lost a good deal of blood, and the placenta was not delivered for some hours. I saw no reason to doubt the truthfulness of the woman's story, and the baby presented its own evidence in the form of a large bruise on the side of the head, another on the shoulder and a third on the right knee. It had probably fallen between the ties on the sand and clear of the rail, which I found, on examination of the hole in the closet was quite possible.

The report met with immediate and persisting skepticism. Published biographies of "The Baby on the Tracks" replete with family photos smack of Marlene Yorrick Davis and have done little, if anything, to increase public acceptance of this story.

Another paper that has suffered the same fate as Osler's "baby on the tracks" is a "gloss attributed to the Hippocratic school," the first English text of a group of lost aphorisms translated by S. N. Gano and published in *The Leech* in 1958. As Gano pointed out in his introduction, "the stylistic traits bear strong evidence of genuineness, and the reader cannot fail to be impressed by the conciseness, clarity, and sagacity which are displayed in almost every paragraph."

The aphorisms give new insight into the clinical outlook of the ancient authors:

1. Absence of respiration is a bad sign.
2. It is unfavorable for the patient to be purple, especially if he is also cold. The physician should not promise a cure in such cases.
4. Hemorrhoids are not improved by horseback riding or by riding on an ass.
11. Patients who always wake up on the wrong side should be treated by purges.
13. To pick at the coverlet indicates alienation of the mind, unless the bed contains small fragments of food.
15. Fevers of eighty days where no cause is apparent produce alienation of mind in the physician.
22. Life is short and the art long; patients are inscrutable; their ignorance is impenetrable, and their relatives are impossible.
23. When swarthy patients have a blonde child and a blonde serving maid, the physician should suspect a displacement of humors. I hold that this condition is no more divine than any other.
25. When the spleen is found on the right side, the patient should consider changing physicians.
30. Dislocation of the neck, which has been produced by a rope, cannot be treated with barley water.
40. Where symptoms are severe and protracted, it is good if the patient's relatives are few, and best if they be absent altogether.

Despite a thorough search, I have not been able to document any previous publication of these aphorisms in any language. Nor have I yet found any of them incorporated into any history of medicine. The latter is probably only a matter of time. Textbooks of medical history are always behind the cutting edge of scholarly advancement.

NOTES

Egerton Y. Davis, a.k.a. Sir William Osler, has been the subject of more publications than any other nineteenth- or twentieth-century clinician. Descriptions of his life vary from brief notes to the massive *Life of Sir William Osler*, by Harvey Cushing (Oxford: Clarendon Press, 1925). The notes by Osler referring to E. Y. D. were first published within these two volumes. Shorter articles focus on individual interests of Osler, from his bedside aphorisms to his literary investigations. The history of E. Y. D. is best presented in E. F. Nation's "Osler's Alter Ego" (*Diseases of the Chest* 56:531–537, 1969). N. L. Caroline and H. Schwartz's "Chicken Soup, Rebound and Relapse of Pneumonia: Report of a Case" appeared in the same journal after it had changed names (*Chest* 67:215–216, 1975). Osler's obstetrical interests are discussed in at least two places:

1. Scarlett, E. P. (1962): William Osler: Obstetrician. *Arch. Intern. Med.*, 109:625–627.

2. Rucker, M. P. (1952): Sir William Osler's obstetrical interests. *Bull. Hist. Med.*, 26:153–161.

C. B. Farrar's "Osler's Story of 'The Baby on the Track' " (*Can. Med. Assoc. J.*, 90:781–784, 1964) gives all the details of this story from its inception through the death of the "baby" at age 74. Some of the satires discussed here have been described before as hoaxes. Two of the most entertaining compilations of medical hoaxes are the following:

1. Jarcho, S. (1959): Some hoaxes in the medical literature. *Bull. Hist. Med.*, 33:342–347.

2. Scarlett, M. B. (1964): Some hoaxes in medical history and literature. *Arch. Intern. Med.*, 113:291–296.

Neither R. P. nor S. N. Gano could be contacted for permission to quote their articles from *The Leech*. The editors of *The Leech* were unaware of their present addresses. SIC TRANSIT GLORIA MUNDI.

The Curse of the Evanses

I have drawn your attention to this form of chorea, gentlemen, not that I considered it of any great practical importance to you, but merely as a medical curiosity, and as such it may have some interest.

George Huntington (1872)

Just as it was always a delight to hear a poet read his own poem, so it was a pleasure and privilege to be able to carry away with them the memory of having seen and heard a man who had helped to make medical history.
Charles Dana, on hearing George
Huntington present a paper on
Huntington's chorea (1909)

The prominence of four American doctors among the five who described the disease between 1841 and 1872 reflects the high standard of medical awareness to the New World and the informational value of the English language rather than the geographical prevalence of Huntington's chorea.

George W. Bruyn (1968)

The Curse of the Evanses

Mrs. Evans: And right to the time the pains come on, I prayed Sammy'd be born dead, and Sammy's father prayed, but Sammy was born healthy and smiling, and we just had to love him, and live in fear. He doubled the torment of fear we lived in. And that's what you'd be in for. And Sammy, he'd go the way his father went. And your baby, you'd be bringing it into torment. I tell you it'd be a crime—a crime worse than murder! So you just can't, Nina!

Nina: What do you mean? Why don't you speak plainly? I think you're horrible! Praying your baby would be born dead! That's a lie! You couldn't!

Mrs. Evans: I thought I was plain, but I'll be plainer. Only remember it's a family secret and now you're one of the family. It's the curse on the Evanses. My husband's mother—she was an only child—died in an asylum and her father before her. I know that for a fact. And my husband's sister, Sammy's aunt, she's out of her mind. She lives on the top floor of this house, hasn't been out of her room in years, I've taken care of her. She just sits, doesn't say a word, but she's happy, she laughs to herself a lot, she hasn't a care in the world. But I remember when she was all right, she was always unhappy, she never got married, most people around here were afraid of the Evanses in spite of their being rich for hereabouts. They knew about the craziness going back, I guess, for heaven knows how long. I didn't know about the Evanses until after I'd married my husband. He came to the town I lived in, no one there knew about the Evanses. He didn't tell me until after we were married. He asked me to forgive him, he said he loved me so much he'd have gone mad without me, said I was his only hope of salvation. So I forgave him. I loved him an awful lot. I said to myself, I'll be his salvation—and maybe I could have if we hadn't had Sammy born. My husband kept real well up to then. We'd swore we'd never have children, we never forgot to be careful for two whole years. Then one night we'd both gone to a dance, we'd both had a little punch to drink, just enough to forget—driving home in the moonlight—that moonlight!—such little things at the back of big things!

Nina: I don't believe you and I won't believe you!

Mrs. Evans: My husband, Sammy's father, in spite of all he and I fought against it, he finally gave in to it when Sammy was only eight, he couldn't keep up any more living in fear for Sammy, thinking any minute the curse might get him, every time he was sick, or had a headache, or bumped his head, or started crying, or had a nightmare and screamed, or said something queer like children do naturally. Living like that with that fear is awful torment! I know that! I went through it by his side! It nearly drove me crazy, too—but I didn't have it in my blood! And that's why I'm telling you! You got to see you can't, Nina!

Nina: I don't believe you! I don't believe Sam would ever have married me if he knew—!

Mrs. Evans: Who said Sammy knew? He don't know a single thing about it! That's been the work of my life, keeping him from knowing.

In this interchange from Act 3 of Eugene O'Neill's play *Strange Interlude* (1928), Huntington's chorea made its stage debut. This scene, in which Mrs. Evans first tells her pregnant daughter-in-law Nina of the dominantly inherited middle-adult-life-onset insanity that runs in the Evans family, has its roots not in literature but in the sufferings of families with Huntington's chorea. Whether or not Eugene O'Neill was fully aware of all the medical and genetic implications of this disease, he certainly understood its emotional effect on families that carry this gene. Such poignant scenes, in which the issue of genetic risk is presented to an outsider who has married into a family with Huntington's chorea, are still being played out today. There are some differences. The risks can now be statistically defined, both for the proband and for any potential children. But the emotional meaning has not changed.

It has now been over 100 years since George Huntington wrote his original paper and put American neurology on the map with a disease of its own. Today Huntington is considered to be one of the founders of American neurology, but he was not a neurologist.

George Summner Huntington (1850–1916) was born in East Hampton, Long Island, New York. His family had been in America for over 200 years, and they traced their descent from Simon Huntington of Norwich, England, who with his wife Margaret Baret and children sailed to America in 1633. In 1797 Dr. Abel Huntington (our Dr. Huntington's grandfather) settled in East Hampton, Long Island, and soon became the leading physician in the region. He was well known as the first physician on Long Island to perform a lithotomy.

Abel Huntington was one of the first physicians in America to take advantage of Jenner's discovery that cowpox vaccination prevented smallpox. He personally prepared and preserved variola virus for vaccination and was in charge of a retreat for those who had been inoculated. He was active in civic affairs as well as medical affairs; he was a presidential elector in 1820 and a New York state senator in 1821. He served two terms as congressman during the administration of Andrew Jackson and even enjoyed the friendship of Old Hickory. In 1845 he was appointed collector of customs for Sag Harbor, and in 1846 he was a member of the committee to revise the constitution of the state of New York.

George Lee Huntington, the only son of Abel Huntington and the father of Dr. George Huntington, was born in East Hampton, L.I., July 15, 1811. He studied medicine with his father, and after receiving his degree from New York University, he joined his father in the practice of medicine in East Hampton. He remained there for the rest of his life.

George Huntington first studied medicine as a sort of apprentice with his father and then graduated from the College of Physicians and Surgeons of Columbia University in the spring of 1871. His graduation thesis was entitled "Opium." After obtaining his medical degree he returned to East Hampton and assisted his father in practice. On Long Island he was able to observe patients with hereditary chorea who had been followed by his family for several generations. Later that year he moved to Pomeroy, Ohio, and on February 15, 1872, he presented a paper entitled "On Chorea" before the Meigs and Mason Academy of Medicine at Middleport, Ohio. It was later published in *The Medical and Surgical Reporter* (26:317–321, 1872):

ON CHOREA

By George Huntington, M.D., of Pomeroy, Ohio

And now I wish to draw your attention more particularly to a form of the disease which exists, so far as I know, almost exclusively on the east end of Long Island. It is peculiar in itself and seems to obey certain fixed laws. In the first place, let me remark that chorea, as it is commonly known to the profession, and a description of which I have already given, is of exceeding rare occurrence there. I do not remember a single instance occurring in my father's practice, and I have often heard him say that it was a rare disease and seldom met with by him.

The hereditary chorea, as I shall call it, is confined to certain and fortunately a few families, and has been transmitted to them, an heirloom from generations away back in the dim past. It is spoken of by those in whose veins the seeds of the disease are known to exist, with a kind of horror, and not at all alluded to except through dire necessity, when it is mentioned as "that disorder." It is attended generally by all the symptoms of common chorea, only in an aggravated degree, hardly ever manifesting itself until adult or middle life, and then coming on gradually but surely, increasing by degrees, and often occupying years in its development, until the hapless sufferer is but a quivering wreck of his former self.

It is common and is indeed, I believe, more common among men than women, while I am not aware that season or complexion has any influence in the matter. There are three marked peculiarities in this disease: 1. Its hereditary nature. 2. A tendency to insanity and suicide. 3. Its manifesting itself as a grave disease only in adult life.

1. Of its hereditary nature. When either or both parents have shown manifestations of the disease, and more especially when these manifestations have been of a serious nature, one or more of the offspring almost invariably suffer from the disease, if they live to adult age. But if by any chance these children go through life without it, the thread is broken and the grandchildren and great grandchildren of the original shakers may rest assured that they are free from the disease. This you will perceive differs from the general laws of so called hereditary diseases, as for instance in phthisis, or syphillis, when one generation may enjoy entire immunity from their dread ravages, and yet in another you find them cropping out in all their hideousness. Unstable and whimsical as the disease may be in other respects in this it is firm, it never skips a generation to again manifest itself in another; once having yielded its claims, it never regains them. In all the families, or nearly all in which the choreic taint exists, the nervous temperament greatly preponderates, and in my grandfather's and father's experience, which conjointly cover a period of 78 years, nervous excitement in a marked degree almost invariably attends upon every disease these people may suffer from, although they may not when in health be over nervous.

2. The tendency to insanity, and sometimes that form of insanity which leads to suicide, is marked. I know of several instances of suicide of people suffering from this form of chorea, or who belonged to families in which the disease existed. As the disease progresses the mind becomes more or less impaired, in many amounting to insanity, while in others mind and body both gradually fail until death relieves them of their sufferings. At present, I know of two married men, whose wives are living, and who are making love to some young lady, not seeming to be aware that there is any impropriety in it. They are suffering from chorea to such an extent that they can hardly walk, and would be thought, by a stranger, to

be intoxicated. They are men of about 50 years of age, but never let an opportunity to flirt with a girl go past unimproved. The effect is ridiculous in the extreme.

3. Its third peculiarity is its coming on, at least as a grave disease, only in the adult life. I do not know of a single case that has shown any marked signs of chorea before the age of thirty or forty years, while those who pass the fortieth year without symptoms of the disease, are seldom attacked. It begins as an ordinary chorea might begin, by the irregular and spasmodic action of certain muscles, as of the face, arms, etc. These movements gradually increase, when muscles hitherto unaffected take on the spasmodic action, until every muscle in the body becomes affected (excepting the involuntary ones), and the poor patient presents a spectacle which is anything but pleasing to witness. I have never known a recovery or even an amelioration of symptoms in this form of chorea; when once it begins it clings to the bitter end. No treatment seems to be of any avail, and indeed nowadays its end is so well known to the sufferer and his friends, that medical advice is seldom sought. It seems at least to be one of the incurables.

Dr. Wood, in his work on the practice of medicine, mentions the case of a man, in the Pennsylvania Hospital, suffering from aggravated chorea, which resisted all treatment. He finally left the hospital uncured. I strongly suspect that this man belonged to one of the families in which hereditary chorea existed. I know nothing of its pathology. I have drawn your attention to this form of chorea gentlemen, not that I considered it of any great practical importance to you, but merely as a medical curiosity, and as such it may have some interest.

In this brief paper, George Huntington clearly delineated the disease that now bears his name. He described its adult onset and its associated behavioral changes, and he observed the results of a mendelian dominant gene long before any of Mendel's work had reached the English-reading world. The great William Osler wrote of this paper: "In the history of medicine there are few instances in which a disease has been more accurately, more graphically, or more briefly described."

Unfortunately, George Huntington found Pomeroy abundantly supplied with physicians, and as the chance for successful practice seemed small, he returned to East Hampton. Then, in 1874, he settled in La Grangeville, Duchess County, New York, where he remained until 1901, when ill health compelled him to go to Asheville, North Carolina. He remained in Asheville for only 2 years and then returned to Duchess County, where he continued to practice until the year before his death. He made no other scientific contribution and never practiced neurology, but he always retained his interest in the medical curiosity he had described in 1872. In a speech before the New York Neurological Society in 1909 he told of his recollections of Huntington's chorea and acknowledged his debt to his father and grandfather. This paper was later published in the *Journal of Nervous and Mental Diseases* (37:255–257, 1910) with the title "Recollections of Huntington's Chorea as I Saw It at East Hampton, Long Island, during my Boyhood."

Huntington prefaced his remarks with the statement that he had seen practically no cases of Huntington's chorea during the long period that had passed since the presentation of his original paper 37 years earlier and that without the facts and observations handed down to him by his grandfather, Dr. Abel Huntington, and his father, Dr. George Lee Huntington, whose medical lives were spent in East

Hampton, L.I., he could never have formulated a picture of the salient characteristics of the disease so true and so complete as to make of it a so-called classic.

Old East Hampton was settled by the English in the year 1649 and was first called Maidstone, after the former home of many of them in England. They had spread eastward from Southampton, whither they had come from New England, principally from Saybrook and its vicinity in Connecticut, and settled several years prior to the settlement in East Hampton. With these earliest settlers, in all probability, came the disease. When Huntington's grandfather came to eastern Long Island from Connecticut in 1797, he found the disease well established there, but he had little or no call to treat it, although he undoubtedly treated many choreics for intercurrent disease and thus was more or less intimately acquainted with them. The same was true of his father, who was a native of East Hampton. Years of contact with these people taught the Huntingtons their peculiarities: the age at which the disease generally manifested itself; its usually slow onset and gradual development, sometimes through a long life, sometimes for only a short period, for many of these people ended it all by suicide before its worst features had time to develop. Some worked at their trades long after the choreic features had developed, but they gradually succumbed to the inevitable, becoming more and more helpless as time advanced, and often mind and body failed with even pace.

In his speech, Huntington said that he believed that the postulates taken in his original paper still held good, namely: the appearance of the disease only in adult life, its chronicity and gradual advancement, its direct line from parent to offspring, and, when this line was broken, its failure to reappear in later generations. Speaking of his personal memories of this form of chorea, Huntington related the following:

> Over fifty years ago, in riding with my father on his professional rounds, I saw my first cases of "that disorder," which was the way in which the natives always referred to the dreaded disease. I recall it as vividly as though it had occurred but yesterday. It made a most enduring impression upon my boyish mind, an impression every detail of which I recall today, an impression which was the very first impulse to my choosing chorea as my virgin contribution to medical lore. Driving with my father through a wooded road leading from East Hampton to Amagansett, we suddenly came upon two women, mother and daughter, both tall, thin, almost cadaverous, both bowing, twisting, grimacing. I stared in wonderment, almost in fear. What could it mean? My father paused to speak with them and we passed on. Then my Gamaliel-like instruction began: my medical education had its inception. From this point on my interest in the disease has never wholly ceased.

In the discussion of this paper, Charles Dana, an eminent neurologist, remarked that Huntington's chorea had always appealed to him as an excellent disease in which to work out and apply the mendelian theory of heredity.

In his own lifetime, George Huntington, a rural general practitioner, had seen his name used eponymously because he had been the first to describe the disease. But had he really been first? Although there had been occasional mentions of adult-onset chorea in the medical literature, the first full description of hereditary chronic chorea in adults was written by Charles O. Waters. Waters was both a physician and a minister. He was born at Franklin, New York, in the western Catskills in

1816. In 1834 he entered Williams College, but he had to leave school before receiving a degree because of several hemorrhages of the lung. In 1839 he entered the medical department of Columbian University in Washington, D.C. Waters described his admission in these words: "At that time, and under a rule of the institution, each Senator of the United States could select a student for one gratuitous course of medical lectures, and I was there as the protege of the Hon. Silas Wright, then one of the Senators from New York." Waters later moved to Philadelphia and graduated from Jefferson Medical College in 1841. He never practiced medicine in the East. After graduation he went West and finally settled in Muscatine, Iowa, where he quietly practiced medicine for over 20 years. He formally entered the Presbyterian ministry in 1860 and thereafter did not practice medicine. At some time in the 1860s he moved to Chicago. His home was lost in the great Chicago fire of 1871. In Chicago he became an elder in the Jefferson Presbyterian Church and in 1880 a trustee of the Chicago Theological Seminary. He died in 1892 of chronic Bright's disease. Although he wrote numerous religious articles and from 1859 to 1892 was a regular contributor to *The Presbyterian*, his contribution to medical science consisted of exactly one letter.

In May, 1841, shortly after his graduation from Jefferson Medical College, Waters wrote his professor of medicine, Robley Dunglison, concerning "the nature of a singular convulsive affection, which, he affirmed, prevailed in a part of the country with which he was familiar." Dunglison, who was not at all familiar with the disorder, printed Waters's letter in the first edition of his book *The Practice of Medicine* (Philadelphia: Lea and Blanchard, 1842):

Franklin, New York, 5th May, 1841.

Prof. R. Dunglison.
Dear Sir:—In obedience to your kind request I improve my first leisure since my return home, in giving you, in as lucid and satisfactory a manner as possible, an account of a singular affection somewhat common in the southeastern portion of this state, and known among the common people as "the magrums." Whence the name originated I know not, but if it be a corruption of the word "megrim," I am at a loss to understand how it ever came to be applied by the vulgar to the disease of which I am speaking, and which has nothing in it analogous to ordinary hemicrania or megrim. It consists essentially in a spasmodic action of all, or nearly all, the voluntary muscles of the system—of involuntary and more or less irregular motions of the extremities, face and trunk. In these involuntary movements the upper part of the air passages occasionally participate, as it is witnessed by the "clucking" sound in the neighborhood of the glottis, and in a manifest impediment to the powers of speech. The expression of countenance, and general appearance of the patient are very much such as are described as characteristic of chorea.
The disease is markedly hereditary, and is most common among the lower classes, though cases of it are not unfrequently found among those, who by industry and temperance have raised themselves to a respectable rank in society. These involuntary movements of the face, neck, extremities and body, cease entirely during sleep.
This singular disease rarely—very rarely indeed—makes its appearance before adult life: and attacks after forty-five years of age are also very rare. When once

it has appeared, however, it clings to the suffering victim with unrelenting tenacity till death comes to his relief. It very rarely or never ceases while life lasts.

The first indications of its approach are spasmodic twitchings of the extremities—generally the fingers—which gradually extend and involve all the voluntary muscles. This derangement of muscular action is by no means uniform: in some it exists to a greater, in others to a less extent, but in all cases it gradually induces a state of more or less perfect dementia.

This disease, in its origin and progress, is not, as far as I have been able to discover, attended with any unusual pain in the head. In some of the worst cases I ever saw, I could not discover, that there had ever been any unusual sensation in the cerebral region.

When speaking of the manifestly hereditary nature of the disease, I should perhaps have remarked, that I have never known a case of it to occur in a patient, one or both of whose ancestors were not, within the third generation at farthest, the subjects of this distressing malady.

The appetite is commonly good, and the process of digestion seems generally to proceed with considerable regularity. The bowels are, however, usually somewhat costive, though I have known cases in which daily evacuations were not unfrequent. Of the general appearance of these evacuations I am not informed.

The pulse does not deviate materially from the healthy standard, and consequently presents nothing remarkable.

It may not be amiss to state, that the last patient who came under my observation, and who had the reputation of being an honest man, informed me, that, in his own case, this involuntary action of the muscles ceased under the influence of all instrumental music, except that of the common "Jew's-Harp." I very much regret that it was not in my power to test the truth of this statement.

I also regret, that it is not now in my power to give any information as to the condition of the catamenia in those labouring under it. I hope to be able to institute a course of inquiry upon this subject during the ensuing summer and fall.

I have thus, dear sir, given you a general—though perhaps not very lucid and satisfactory—account of this singular malady. I may observe that, although no descriptions of chorea in the books apply very well to this disease, it nevertheless seems to differ in several respects from ordinary chorea. 1st. It rarely occurs before adult age. 2nd. It never ceases spontaneously. 3rd. When fully developed it wants the paroxysmal character.

After all, may not this disease be a peculiar modification of chorea?—is not its pathology in the main the same, and would it not probably be found to yield to the treatment suited to chorea, if to any?

I am, dear sir, respectfully,
Your ob't serv't,

C. O. Waters

This letter produced some interest in adult-onset chorea in the United States, and the third edition of Dunglison's *The Practice of Medicine* (1848) contained another reference to such disorders by Charles Rollins Gorman.

Gorman was born August 4, 1817, at Barkhamsted, Connecticut. His father was Dr. James T. Gorman, who at some time in middle life moved with his family from Connecticut to Benton, Pennsylvania, where he practiced until his death in 1861. It is thus evident that the younger Gorman, like Huntington, had the advantage of medical ancestry in preparing his paper.

Charles Gorman's mother was Lois Beecher Gorman, a second cousin of Henry Ward Beecher. He graduated from Jefferson Medical College in 1848. He practiced in Phillipsburg, New Jersey, for 12 or 18 months. He later settled in Pittston, Pennsylvania, where he continued his practice to the time of his death in 1879.

The following note appears in the third edition of Dunglison's *Practice*:

> In an inaugural dissertation, presented before the Faculty of Jefferson Medical College of Philadelphia, by Dr. Charles R. Gorman, of Luzerne County, Pa., the writer states that this affection prevails also in other portions of the country. According to him it seems to be circumscribed by neighborhood boundaries, and to be confined to sections of the country, the inhabitants of which are intimately connected in their social or business relations. "May not this circumstance," he asks, "sanction the inference that the cause exists in the influence of the morals known to exert over the physical—the sympathy of imitation."

It is not possible to trace this paper any further, because Gorman's thesis of 1848 was lost along with much other material when the old college building of Jefferson Medical College was torn down.

A third American description of chorea also appeared prior to Huntington's paper. In 1863, Irving Whitall Lyon, then a house physician at Bellevue Hospital, New York City, published the following report in the *American Medical Times* (7:289, 1863)

> The writer has been familiar from childhood with a type of chorea so unlike in its origin to anything described in our standard textbooks, that the publication of a few facts in relation thereto has been thought advisable, not only as a matter of interest to the reader, but more especially for the purpose of eliciting the observations of any who may have met with indications of kindred significance.
>
> The peculiarity of origin claimed for this type consists in its hereditary transmissibility: this claim we will endeavor to support by the following facts and considerations:—
>
> The disease, as we have been accustomed to observe it, is known in the community by the name of migrims. Of the origin or derivation of the term but little can be ascertained, except the conjecture that it may be a corruption of megrim, which word, to say the least, is very inexpressive of any leading character of the malady, which is chorea in toto, consisting of "irregular action of the voluntary muscles, when stimulated by the will," and marked by an obstinate chronicity.
>
> It is confined almost exclusively to certain families, so that such are popularly denominated the "migrim families;" and the children of parents affected with this disorder are very liable to become the subjects of its manifestations and in turn transmit it in their offspring. So strong is the conviction of its hereditary influence that the people among whom it occurs believe this to constitute its only legitimate method of propagation, and acting accordingly, have repeatedly been known to interdict marriage alliances between their children and those believed to be tainted with the migrim diathesis, under the severe penalties of disinheritance and social ostracism. It is however, regarded by many as a disgraceful disease; for what reason it would be difficult to understand, unless we admit the influence of a tradition that ascribes the ultimate origin of the disease to a visitation upon those who reviled and mimicked our Saviour while undergoing crucifixion, that they and their children were ever after affected with choreal irregularities.
>
> Not only do those exempt from the diathesis insist upon its hereditary nature, but even those in whom the disease is manifest are free to admit the same thing,

and in one instance a gentlemen obligingly volunteered to furnish proof of its existence in his own family for several successive generations.

Aged and very intelligent medical gentlemen, who have practiced for the greater part of their professional lives in communities where the so called migrims prevail, testify that they entertain no doubt of its hereditary communicability.

The author included three case reports and then added the following:

To these cases many more might be added, were they deemed necessary to establish the claim premised; let us briefly recapitulate:

First.—The deep seated popular belief in the hereditary nature of the disease. Such an argument, it may be urged, is unphilosophical, and popular notions of disease should not be accredited by professional men. But such an objection cannot well be urged here, since the truth of the matter can only be arrived at by observation: and as the symptoms of chorea are patent and easy of cognition to all, we conclude the testing of any intelligent observer of this disease to be valid and worthy of credence, whether he be educated in the medical profession or not.

Second.—The above reason derives additional support from the acknowledgements of those affected with the disease, for it must be a thorough conviction, that would lead a person to avow a hereditary vice of constitution, which is at once injurious to his reputation and prospects in life: and

Third.—The supposed objections to the first answered, and it together with the second reason substantiated by the testimony of medical men conversant with the disease. So much for the moral; now for the demonstrative evidence.

We have cited one instance in which chorea was shown to have occurred in a family throughout five successive generations, and in different persons of the same generation; this is a phenomenon too remarkable to be explained in any other way than the one proposed, and although the second and third cases do not go so far, still they cannot mean anything less than what is claimed for the first case. It may be well to state, in this connexion, that the advantages for investigating the last two cases were not such as would enable us to decide whether the disease could be traced further back or not. . . .

In conclusion, we would again invite the publication of any facts which may assist in elucidating this subject, for it certainly is one of real interest; and as we know that many physicians are daily observing just what has been described, we are confident that some new and acceptable offering will be made from such sources.

Irving Lyon was born October 18, 1840, at Bedford, Westchester County, New York. His father was Solomon R. Lyon, a ruling elder in the local Presbyterian church. He received his M.D. from the University of Vermont in 1862 and from the College of Physicians and Surgeons, New York, in 1863.

He was an acting assistant surgeon early in the Civil War, and he became demonstrator of anatomy in the famous Berkshire Medical School in 1862. He served as a member of the house staff of Bellevue Hospital in 1863 and 1864. In the fall of 1864 he settled in Hartford, Connecticut, and practiced there until his death in 1896. Thus it appears possible that three other American physicians described chronic hereditary adult chorea before Huntington did. But was it Huntington's chorea? In 1908 there was a special Huntington number of the periodical *Neurographs* (1:137–149). In this, the editor, William Browning, Ph.B., M.D., raised the same question and tried to trace the patients seen by Waters, Gorman, and Lyon to answer the question.

In his original letter, Waters wrote that the "singular affection" he was describing was "common in the southeastern portion of the state" (New York). This, Browning believed, suggested that Waters was referring to East Hampton, Long Island, but on careful investigation it appeared that he meant Westchester County, the source of Lyon's cases. In this same report, Browning demonstrated that Lyon's patients had Huntington's chorea. Lyon's article began as follows: "The writer has been familiar from childhood with a type of chorea so unlike in its origin to anything described in our standard text-books." Although he avoided specifying the region of his cases more exactly, even dating his article Bellevue Hospital, he did note that two were in the state of New York and one in Connecticut. Lyon was born at Bedford, Westchester County, New York, adjoining the western boundary of Connecticut; he spent his boyhood there and made that his home until taking his medical degree. It seems evident that his observations were made in that region. This is the region where the disorder was called "magrums," a phenomenon also reported by Waters, and this corroborated the identity of the two patient populations. Bedford is well known as a locale with a high incidence of Huntington's chorea.

Browning was also able to report on Gorman's patients. He believed that Gorman's patients were from Pennsylvania. In 1889 Sinkler wrote an article in the *Journal of Nervous and Mental Disease* in which he presented a family history of patients with Huntington's chorea from Nicholson, Pennsylvania. This town directly adjoins Benton in Lackawanna County, the place where Gorman's father practiced medicine and where Gorman naturally spent much time in his younger years and did his medical apprenticeship. It thus appears that Waters, Gorman, and Lyon did describe what turned out to be Huntington's chorea. Why, then, is it called Huntington's chorea? Certainly Huntington's description was more complete, and, more important, it was published at the right time to catch the imagination of early clinical neurologists. Huntington's paper, unlike the previous reports, was abstracted into German by Kussmaul and Nothnagel, and soon the eponym was born.

These families can be traced back much further than Browning imagined, back to 1630 and even before. In the 1630s there was considerable turmoil in England. Charles I had been king for 5 years. He continued his father's policy of harrying nonconformists out of the land. Under Charles I, Archbishop Laud increased the vigor with which the Church of England persecuted religious nonconformists. The nonconformists and Puritans, as a result of such harassment, were leaving England as quickly as they could find ships to transport them. In 1630 a well-known fleet led by John Winthrop left England for America with about 700 passengers.

These immigrants included a number of residents from the small village of Bures in Suffolk, England. Three men and their wives in this group seem to have brought chorea to America in their search for religious freedom. The romantic view of American history relates that the founding fathers, always pictured as Puritans, came to America to avoid religious persecution. However, pursuit of religious freedom by nonconformists was not the only reason to leave England, and Puritans were not the only English citizens being persecuted. At that time in England (and also, unfortunately, in the English colonies in the New World) it was a religious duty to seek out and destroy all of those who were believed to have a secret compact with the Prince of Hell. In Bures and vicinity the Church of England was very active in this pursuit, zealously demolishing so-called superstitious ornaments in nonconformist churches. Witch-hunters assisted by bell-ringers canvassed the country and received 20 shillings from the government for every suspected witch who was jailed. Only accusation, not conviction, was required before the witch-hunters could receive their reward. Witchcraft was a deadly sin, and hundreds of odd and unpopular citizens were tortured and executed as enemies of mankind. Witchcraft and accusations of being a practicing witch were not the only threats to the populace. The English penal code was merciless in its punishment of civil and criminal offences. Those convicted of various crimes often accepted banishment to the colonies in order to avoid jail.

The fundamental beliefs about witchcraft in Connecticut and the other New England colonies were the same as those in England. Each witch scare began with the discovery that a certain person within the community, almost invariably an adult woman, had taken on "spectral" changes in her appearance and actions. These alterations in conduct were viewed with suspicion by neighbors as evidence of familiarity with the devil, and subsequently they were reported to the authorities. The occurrence of these "spectral" changes meant that the devil had already approached, seduced, and embraced the woman. The woman, in turn, had weakened under the devil's promises to defend her and finally had signed a covenant with the devil in her own blood. In this covenant, the woman gave her body and soul to the devil and thereby had forsaken both God and the church. This was a common belief of the populace, but it was very seldom admitted by the accused witch, except during torture.

The devil was believed to visit the witch at night to consort with her. While consorting, the devil would claw and scratch her, leaving conspicuous marks on her skin. She then would develop nipples in these sites of injury; these were for imps to suckle on. These imps usually attached themselves to her body, often hanging from her breasts and genitals.

Witch-hunts may well have been one of the factors that forced families with Huntington's chorea to leave England. But merely crossing an ocean was not sufficient to escape persecution.

It appears that among the first to bring Huntington's chorea to the New World were two half-brothers, Geoffrey and Nicholas Haste, and one William Knapp. Geoffrey Haste was a member of the Court of Ferrier of Bures, and when his family objected to his chosen bride because her lineage could not be traced back to Norman times, Geoffrey and his wife-to-be fled to America, where they finally settled in Stamford, Connecticut. Once settled, Geoffrey distinguished himself in various colonial criminal records by signing, along with others, harsh verdicts on his fellow colonists. One of these cases involved a man who was held responsible for the pregnancy of a young woman. He was sentenced to stand on the pillory to be publicly whipped and to have the letter R burned on his cheek; he was to pay the young woman's parents 10 pounds, and he was to marry her as soon as he recovered. In spite of the woman's low morals, as brought out in later proceedings, the verdict stood. Such extreme forms of punishment were popular in those days. Geoffrey Haste himself was fined in court for questioning testimony against him, and on another occasion he was accused in court of retaining a stolen calf. His eldest son faced a death sentence on a charge of "bestialitie," but the magistrate decreased the sentence to two severe public whippings, a fine, and a halter to be fastened on his neck, which he was compelled to wear in public for 2 years. Following this punishment, the son became quite religious; he moved to another state, and many of his direct descendants became afflicted with adult chorea.

Another of Geoffrey's sons showed his suceptibility to the religious insanity of the day by acting as a juryman in the trial of Mercy Disborough for witchcraft and finding her guilty. His descendants did not demonstrate chorea. At least one other son gave birth to a long line of choreatic individuals, but yet another son, known in the neurologic literature by the name of Jefferson, deserves particular attention. He was one of the first settlers in Greenwich, Connecticut, a community that was not in sympathy with the spirit of the Puritans. This settlement, on the border of the Dutch and Puritan settlements, served as a retreat for immoral, treacherous, and vicious men. In 1655 the deputies in neighboring Stamford complained to the general court at New Haven about intolerable drunkenness among the English and the Indians in Greenwich, maintaining that the inhabitants were harboring runaway servants and that marriages in the community were often irregular. In the next year, Jefferson, with a few other settlers, signed an agreement in court to yield themselves up to the lawful authorities. He later became a deputy for several years, and he retired from public life at the age of 44 years. He was ill for some time before his death at the age of 61 years. Jefferson married the daughter of Nicholas, his father's half-brother. From this marriage at least 10 generations of known choreics have sprung.

Nicholas Haste himself was not without problems. He brought his wife Ellin with him from Bures, England, in the Winthrop fleet. The passengers on these ships had suffered from scurvy and malnutrition, as had many of those who previously traveled the Atlantic on the Mayflower. John Winthrop, the Puritan leader who commanded this fleet, described in his log the hunger and disease that quickly thinned out the ranks of potential settlers. On landing, Nicholas was brought before the magistrates of the community for his actions during the arduous journey. He apparently had seized on the deprivations of the long voyage as an opportunity to line his own pockets. Their estimate of this quack was obviously very low, for he "was fined by the court 5 pounds for taking upon him to cure the scurvy by a water of no value, which he sold to a very dear rate; to be imprisoned till he pay his fine, or give security for it, or else be whipped and be liable to any man's action of whom he had received for said water." His wife Ellin, the mother of Jefferson's wife, was tried for witchcraft in 1653. She was found guilty and hanged.

Just before Ellin was to be hanged for witchcraft, she stepped down dramatically from the scaffold and whispered in the ear of Roger Ludlow, the deputy governor of Massachusetts and Connecticut. After she was cut down, she was examined by several women for devil's nipples and other anatomic evidence of her relationship with Satan. Among these women was a Mary Staplies, who had the courage to speak out and say that she had found no "witches teates" and to further declare that if Ellin was guilty, then she too was a witch. What relationship, if any, this fearless young woman bore to Ellin cannot be ascertained from records, but Roger Ludlow quickly retaliated and proclaimed that Ellin had whispered that Mary Staplies was a witch. The young woman's husband thereupon brought a lawsuit against Roger Ludlow for slander and won a verdict of 15 pounds. In 1654 Mary Staplies was acquitted. Later, in 1692, she and her daughter, Mary Harvey, and grand-daughter, Hannah Harvey, were tried and acquitted of witchcraft. In the trial of Mary Staplies, strange gymnastic performances and peculiar movements were attributed to Mary by a witness.

One of Nicholas and Ellin's granddaughters, Mercy Disborough, was tried twice in the witch-mania epidemic of 1692 for that same capital offense. She was finally pardoned by the justices as the craze ran its course and the authorities, perhaps out of remorse, began reversing previous decisions. One of their sons gave rise to a family carrying the Huntington gene. The same happened to the family of their daughter and Jefferson. It is generally believed that Geoffrey and Ellin themselves had Huntington's chorea. It is less clear that Jefferson was affected.

The third affected family was that of William Knapp. After landing in Boston Bay, William was taken to court to meet Sir Richard Saltonstall, a slaveowner and bondholder, and it was pronounced that all future employers of William must pay Sir Richard one-half of William's wages until he had been reimbursed some 19 pounds. It is not known if this bond was negotiated by the ship captain as payment for transportation or if it had a more pejorative basis. In any case, William and his sons were notorious principals in some of the less savory aspects of colonial life. During the first 10 years after his landing, the records of Massachusetts reveal several arrests. For public profanity, he had to furnish bond for 10 pounds, pending trial. For selling beer for 2 years without a license, he was fined 5 pounds. On another occasion, a payment of 100 pounds and imprisonment were mentioned for making an offensive speech against Governor John Winthrop, who was then insisting on law and order in Massachusetts. In 1643 his wife Elizabeth Warne was mistress of a licensed "house of entertainment" in Boston, and in the following year there was another record of a fine of 5 pounds against William. A daughter of William and Elizabeth married a man named Mulfoot (later changed to Mulford) and moved to East Hampton, Long Island, forming the parent stem of what proved to be the historic Long Island group of Huntington's chorea.

William's eldest son and his wife Priscilla were taken into custody in 1641 and charged with "distemper." Later on, this same son stole some of his mother's family silver, and the court compelled him to return it. In general, William Knapp's children were not tolerated and were publicly warned against settlement in certain parts of the colony.

William Knapp and Elizabeth Warne had another daughter named Elizabeth Knapp. In her early adult life this young woman achieved great notoriety as the celebrated Groton witch. Not only did William have children with Huntington's chorea; Elizabeth Warne may also have had the gene. Following her husband's early death, Elizabeth Warne left her daughter Elizabeth Knapp; she sailed back to England and settled in Suffolk, where she was later accused of being possessed of the devil, was arrested, and even confessed to witchcraft. In the files of the British Museum, records of the complaint brought against Elizabeth Warne by one John Buttery can still be found. In these, Buttery swore that a child developed strange convulsions because of Elizabeth. The guards watched Elizabeth for 3 days and nights for evidence of witchcraft, at the end of which time she is said to have confessed that "she had the devil within her body" and asked that she be punished. Although there were hundreds accused of witchcraft in Suffolk in the seventeenth century, the county records give few details. Unfortunately, there are very few accurate historical documents of witch trials held in England before 1690. It is of interest that affected Warne (Warren) descendants can still be found in the Boston area.

Like her mother in England, Elizabeth Knapp was accused of witchcraft. In 1671 the Reverend Samuel Willard, who was then minister of Groton, wrote a letter to Cotton Mather in which he described the younger Elizabeth's peculiar behavior:

> This poore & miserable object, about a fortnight before shee was taken, wee observed to carry herselfe in a strange & unwonted manner, sometimes shee would give sudden shriekes, & if wee enquired a Reason, would alwayes put it off with some excuse, & then would burst forth into imoderate & extravagant laughter, in such wise, as some times shee fell onto ye ground with it: I myselfe observed oftentimes a strange change in here countenance, but could not suspect ye true reason, but conceived shee might bee ill, and therefore divers times enquired how shee did it, & shee alwayes answered well; which made mee wonder.

Several days later her abnormal behavior worsened:

> ye rest of ye family being in bed, shee was . . . suddenly throne downe into ye midst of ye floore with violence, & taken with a violent fit, whereupon ye whole family was raised, & with much adoe was she kept out of ye fire from destroying her selfe after which time she was followed with fits from thence till ye sabbath day; in which she was violent with bodily motions, leapings, strainings & strange agitations, scarce to be held in bounds by the strength of 3 or 4: violent alsoe in roarings & screamings, representing a dark resemblance of hellish torm, and frequently using in these fits divers words, sometimes crying out money, money, sometimes, sin & misery with other words.

Reverend Willard, doing his duty as he saw it, questioned Elizabeth about her relationship with Satan. Under his questioning she admitted that she had been receiving visits from Satan for 3 years and that he was continuing to torment her. Her consulting physician concluded that she had "Distemper" that was "Diabolicall" in origin. Whether Elizabeth actually had "Diabolicall Distemper," hysteria, or overt Huntington's chorea remains unclear, but her father was choreatic, and her mother also came from choreatic stock.

Certainly not all of the New England witches had Huntington's chorea, but seven came from affected families and were at least subjects at risk. Of these, one certainly had abnormal movements that were apparent to her accusers. Of course, not all Huntington families can be traced to these three families. Another group can be traced back to France, and their story has a familiar ring. In 1685 the Edict of Nantes was revoked, and religious tolerance in France came to an abrupt end. Many Huguenots fled France to avoid fanatic religious persecution. Some came to Halifax, Nova Scotia, and brought Huntington's chorea with them. Other families with chorea have come from Germany, Ireland, and other European countries, including even Norway. This is perhaps the most interesting group, because Norway is the only country in which hereditary chorea was known and described prior to George Huntington's paper.

In 1859, 1860, and 1868 a Norwegian physician named Lund wrote three papers on hereditary chorea in two families of the Bygland and Valle parishes in Saetesdal, Norway. Lund presented a complete picture of Huntington's chorea. He reported that the disease was known as *rykka* (twitches) and was known to be inherited. Lund described its insidious onset between the ages of 50 and 60, its progressive course leading to dementia, and the absence of twitches during sleep. The last fact was not observed by Huntington. In a brief addendum to the 1868 report, Knud Hedd of Tysstad, a farmer, related that the disease usually began in the 30s and resulted in death between the ages of 40 and 50. In later work, the Norwegian Valle pedigree has been traced back to 1550, and new cases descended from these patients continue to appear. Had Lund only had the foresight to write in English rather than Norwegian, today his name might be an eponym or at least part of a hyphenated one.

NOTES

The 1908 Huntington's number of *Neurographs* remains the best source for information on the early history of Huntington's chorea, its describers, and its sufferers. Both Russel DeJong's "George Huntington and His Relationship to the Earlier Description of Chronic Hereditary Chorea" (*Annals of Medical History* 9:201–210, 1937) and Andre Barbeau's "The Understanding of Involuntary Movements: An Historical Approach" (*Journal of Nervous and Mental Disease* 127:469–489, 1958) also present some aspects of this story.

The histories of the early New England families and their relationships to the witch trials have been published at least twice previously in more complete detail: P. R. Vessie, "On the Transmission of Huntington's Chorea for 300 Years—The Bures Family Group," *Journal of Nervous and Mental Disease* 76:533–570, 1932; John Terry Maltsberger, "Even unto the Twelfth Generation—Huntington's

Chorea," *Journal of the History of Medicine and Allied Sciences* 1:1–17, 1961. Of the various papers on witchcraft in New England, I have always liked Charles S. Potts's "An Account of the Witch Craze in Salem with Reference to Some Modern Witch Crazes" (*Archives of Neurology and Psychiatry* 3:465–484, 1920).

Sir Patrick Manson
and
The Kidnapping of Sun Yat-sen

I regarded medicine as the kindly aunt who would bring me out on the high road of politics.

Sun Yat-sen

Sir Patrick Manson
and
The Kidnapping of Sun Yat-sen

To many Americans, if not most, Sun Yat-sen is a name that is only vaguely recalled. His bronze statue, by a San Francisco sculptor, Beniamino Bufano, can still be found in a quiet park in that city's Chinatown, an enduring if often-ignored tribute to one of the founders of the first ill-fated Republic of China. This physician-politician deserves to be better remembered, as does Sir Patrick Manson. Manson was the father of tropical medicine, but today his name is recognized by even fewer Americans than is the name of Sun Yat-sen. Even among physicians his contributions to science are forgotten, and his singular contribution to political history seems to be a well-kept secret. But at a critical time the lives of Manson and Sun Yat-sen intersected, and Manson was instrumental in saving young Sun Yat-sen's life so that he could live to carry out his political destiny.

Sir Patrick Manson (1844–1922) was born in a small ancient village near Aberdeen, Scotland, into a family of considerable means. His father was a landowner and bank manager, and when Patrick was 13 years of age, the family moved to Aberdeen, which they believed offered better educational opportunities for their children. Patrick, like his siblings, went to the Gymnasium and then the West End Academy. As a student he did not show any special promise. It appears that he was considerably more fond of carpentry, hunting, and mechanics than of formal education. A prophetic but most likely apocryphal story is told that while still in his early teens Patrick shot a cat on his father's farm, dissected it, and became fascinated by the tapeworms he encountered during the dissection. If this tale is to be believed, this event determined his life work. At the age of 15 he quit school and was apprenticed in the ironworks of his mother's family, where he was shown little favoritism and carried out the same heavy labor as the other workmen. While in the metalworks he developed what was described as a flaccid paralysis of his right arm. This has been attributed by most biographers to an associated scoliosis, which seems unlikely, and by others to lead poisoning. Although the cause of this disorder is not known, its course and effects are. His arm improved partially, but some weakness remained throughout his life. The physicians who treated young Patrick advised him to observe modified bed rest for most of each day and to give up all hard physical labor. While following this routine, Manson spent most of his time reading natural history, and as a result he developed an interest in medicine. When, after some 5 months of confinement, he was finally allowed to resume his life, he decided to study medicine. Toward this end, Patrick entered the University of Aberdeen in 1860 and complemented these studies with work at Edinburgh University during the summer.

He obtained his M.B. and C.M. degrees at Aberdeen and soon after was appointed assistant medical officer at the Durham lunatic asylum. While working at Durham, he performed numerous postmortem examinations and prepared his thesis, "A Peculiar Affection of the Internal Carotid Artery in Connection with Diseases of the Brain." As a result of this work he was awarded his M.D. at Aberdeen in 1866. Once he had completed his thesis, his interest in working at the asylum quickly waned, and he looked elsewhere for employment and adventure. The opportunities of the British Empire beckoned to him, and he obtained an appointment to the Chinese imperial maritime customs service as medical officer for Formosa.

In June, 1866, he arrived at Takao, Formosa. His professional life in Formosa had two separate parts: his official duties, which included care of patients in the mission hospital, and his private practice. This latter obviously went well, for in only 4 years he was able to repay his father the £700 his medical education had cost. While he was in Formosa he suffered his first acute attack of gout, a malady that was to be a serious handicap to him throughout his life. In 1871, political unrest on the island forced him to transfer to another post within the Chinese imperial maritime customs system.

A new position was found at Amoy, where he filled much the same sort of post as in Formosa. This Chinese city, with a population then of 300,000 Chinese and about 280 foreigners, is on an island some 300 miles north of Hong Kong. The island is only 9 miles in circumference; it lies in the bay of Hiu Tau, and at that time it had two fine harbors that were open to ships of all nations. As a result, it was a very busy place, with a great deal of trade passing through its harbors. The Chinese part of Amoy was filthy and overcrowded, but the Europeans had good housing with plenty of open space.

Manson lived there for 13 years. In addition to his official duties, he was in charge of the mission hospital. Those who practiced Western medicine in China had to overcome many difficulties. Manson found, in Amoy, persistent rumors that a poisonous pill was being distributed by European doctors. He combated this, to some extent, by saying that his hospital provided the antidote free of charge. This solution posed a second problem, because the Chinese did not think much of treatment that could be had for nothing. Manson met this problem by charging those Chinese who could easily afford his services. As a result of his public relations, many who ordinarily would not have gone to a European doctor came to see Manson. Another problem was caused by the fact that the native practitioners worked in the open. They would prescribe in the street, whereas the foreign doctors lured their patients into hidden consulting rooms. Such a closed-door policy led to distrust among the Chinese, who were used to diagnosis and treatment in the open marketplace. Manson's solution was to examine and prescribe for patients in a room that was open to the street. This tended to promote confidence among his Chinese patients. Distrust of doctors who didn't charge and who worked behind closed doors was a minor problem in comparison with the difficulty such a doctor faced in trying to get permission for a post mortem examination. He faced this problem both in his early days in Amoy and later, when his reputation as a physician and research scientist had been established:

One of my filarial patients was dying of an intercurrent disease. Being eager to find the parental form of the filaria, I offered him two hundred dollars to be handed to his widow for permission to perform a postmortem dissection of his body. He agreed, and a proper document was drawn up. . . . On his death the widow claimed the money and I was allowed to dissect the body. My brother and I proceeded to the man's house in the very heart of the native town, prepared to spend several hours in search of the parental filaria then not yet discovered. I had hardly commenced the section when we heard an ominous noise outside. A mob had gathered and was anxious to know what the "foreign devils" were doing. We had to run for our lives and I lost my two hundred dollars.

The only other autopsy I ever had the opportunity of performing on a native was done surreptitiously. The case was one of stricture of the oesophagus and, as this condition is very common in and about Amoy, I was anxious to see the local condition. During the examination I found the Dibothriocephalid larva now called Sparganum mansoni.

The growth of Manson's practice was aided by the fact that his early operations frequently were successful. Many stories of these early successes have been preserved. One involved a young man with marked scrotal enlargement due to elephantiasis. He was totally disabled by this mass. He was unable to work at all and had become a burden to his relatives, who advised him to commit suicide. He tried this three separate times using arsenic. However, he took so much that each time he immediately became nauseated and vomited, thus preventing the poison from working. He was seen by Manson, who advised a surgical procedure to relieve him of the tumor. Apparently he consented to the operation not because he had any confidence in Manson's therapeutic venture but because he believed that the surgeon would be more successful at ending his life than he had been. To the utter amazement of the patient and his relatives, the surgery was successful in relieving the tumor. Manson also performed several successful lithotomies, which greatly impressed the Chinese, who could actually be shown the stones that had been removed.

Manson worked industriously with little help, except for 2 years, when his brother David, who was a missionary doctor, worked with him. He enlarged the hospital, translated Curling's *Diseases of the Testicle* into Chinese, and trained a few Chinese in the ways of Western medicine.

In 1875 he went back to England for some much-deserved rest, relaxation, and rejuvenation. By this time he had amassed a store of practical knowledge in many areas of medicine and surgery. In the latter he had been entirely self-taught. While rummaging in the dusty precincts of the reading room of the British Museum, he chanced upon something that changed his life. There he found the writings of one Timothy Lewis, an officer in the army medical service in India. Lewis, while working in Calcutta, had discovered a minute worm in the blood in several natives he had examined in that city. However, beyond noting it as a curiosity, Lewis had placed no great significance on the observation. With that instinctive insight that afterward became the chief characteristic in his scientific makeup, Manson sought out the connection between this worm, the *Filaria sanguinis-hominis* (the filaria of human blood), and that most disfiguring disease, elephantiasis, that had been such a familiar sight to him in the streets of Amoy. In London and in Edinburgh he familiarized himself with the techniques of the compound microscope, which had then just been introduced as an aid to medical practice; he acquired the best available microscope and returned to his post at Amoy in the early winter of 1875. From that time onward he produced a stream of papers that were printed in the nonmedical pages of reports of the imperial maritime customs service of China. This periodical at that time included the writings of numerous distinguished contributors dealing with many aspects of life in China. It embodied a wealth of information not matched in any similar publication, and it can be used to gauge the work of the British pioneers in the Chinese Empire. It was because of their initial publication in this nonscientific journal that Manson's many medical writings were so slow to be appreciated by the medical profession.

Back in Amoy, his professional life continued to be divided into two separate aspects. First, there were the duties of a medical practitioner, which kept him very busy. He described himself as an indifferent surgeon, but a good carpenter. Nevertheless, in 1877 he performed 237 operations, and in 1879 there were 379. The second aspect of his work consisted of original investigation. His desire to learn about the diseases afflicting his Chinese patients was strong. Indeed, if we consider the obstacles he encountered, it was altogether remarkable. He went to the East very young. He had had no more scientific training than the average young medical student of those days. He had no scientific mentors with whom he could correspond. In such remote places as Formosa and Amoy there was no one with whom he could discuss his findings. He had no means of keeping up with the scientific literature, and he had no real laboratory. His only equipment was his microscope. Yet his accomplishments were brilliant and revolutionary. As a result of his investigations, Manson introduced the concept of transmission of infection by arthropods. This paved the way for a totally new understanding of many diseases.

Manson's most important medical contribution was his successful search for the intermediate host for *Filaria*. The *Filaria* embryos had been detected in human blood by Lewis in 1872. The parent worm was discovered in 1876 by Bancroft, of Brisbane, in whose honor it is now called *Filaria bancrofti*.

Manson observed that the incidence of filariasis in infested areas might be as high as 50% of the population. He found that most of those affected were in apparent good health, despite the finding of parasites in their blood. In other patients who had clinical symptoms, he could not recover the parasite:

> I set to work to ascertain to what extent the population was infected, and for this purpose trained two of my native dressers in blood examinations . . . I remarked that one of the two men who were helping me found very few infected subjects, whilst the other found a much larger number, and I noted that the former did most of his work in the daytime, whilst the other worked in the evening. . . . But thoroughly to establish this, in addition to many shorter observations, a prolonged investigation was undertaken in which blood examinations were made every three hours for six weeks. To do this, I selected two natives who themselves had filaria in their blood, trained them in the use of the microscope and set them to work to examine each other. The result of this examination was conclusive.

He summarized these results as follows:

> You will find that if [*Filaria*] is present in enormous numbers—perhaps three or four hundred per drop—at midnight, that it is practically absent at midday; that it begins to put in an appearance about six or seven in the evening, gradually increasing in numbers up to about midnight and gradually decreasing in numbers up to about seven or eight in the morning and that it is almost entirely absent from eight to nine a.m., till about six or seven p.m.

Only many years later, after he had left China and returned to England, did he discover the site of origin in the body of the filariae that appeared intermittently in the peripheral circulation. The discovery was made at Charing Cross Hospital, where he saw a patient with a small tumor on the arm. After it was removed, in it was found a live female *Filaria bancrofti*, which swam about in normal saline for 12 hours before it died. The patient committed suicide the next morning. At postmortem examination, no embryos were found circulating in the blood, although they had been observed there during the daytime. But after a complete examination, the embryos were found in millions in the capillaries of the lung.

From his discovery of their diurnal appearance in the blood, Manson sought to answer the question of how the filariae entered and left the body. He reasoned as follows:

> The abstracting agency must be a blood-eater or blood-sucker of nocturnal habits, and that it operates through the skin. Further, this blood-sucker of nocturnal habits must have a geographical range corresponding to that of the filaria—that is to say, be indigenous to the tropics and subtropics.

The most likely candidate for this role, Manson believed, was the common tropical mosquito *Culex fatigans*, a hypothesis he soon tested:

> One of my own servants, a Chinese, was infected. On negotiation, he agreed for a large sum, to him, of one dollar to submit to mosquito puncture during an undetermined number of nights. Placing him in a mosquito-curtained enclosure in the evening and, when the number of mosquitoes attracted to the patient by means of a small oil lamp seemed sufficient, I closed the curtain door and left him there till next morning with the attending mosquitoes. Then I collected those mosquitoes which presented abdomens distended with blood, and dissected them, at various periods after they had bitten, by separating with needles the abdomen from the rest of the insects body and had the great satisfaction of finding numerous filariae wriggling actively within their stomachs in the contained inspissating blood.

Despite his discovery of the first arthropod intermediate host, his understanding of the role of the mosquito in spreading disease was far from complete. He erroneously thought that when the mosquito died in water where it had laid eggs, the *Filaria* larvae were set free in the water and from there either were swallowed by humans or actually penetrated the skin by boring through it. It is now known that they are transmitted to humans by the bite of the mosquito. Still, Manson's finding was a great discovery. He had shown, for the first time, that metoxeny, or change of host, occurred between humans and mosquitoes. The full extent of the role of mosquitoes in the spreading of parasitic diseases was soon demonstrated by experimental transmission of a disease of man and lower animals through an intermediary. Theobald Smith, in 1893, furnished the final link in the chain of evidence by infecting healthy cattle with the offending parasite of Texas cattle fever, which he had obtained from the host tick.

Manson's reports on *Filaria* were buried in the customs reports, but some years later he published them in a book, *The Filaria Sanguinis Hominis and Certain New Forms of Parasitic Diseases in India, China and Warm Countries*.

Manson's facilities for research were most limited, and the results he achieved in such conditions are therefore all the more to be admired:

> During this time I investigated a good many other local diseases, but felt the need of books, criticism and medical companionship. Again in the matter of apparatus I was handicapped. No incubator was available until I had manufactured one out of a kerosene tin and a packing-case. Working with some bacterial diseases I had recourse to a sitting fowl as incubator. My cultures, placed in capillary tubes, were sealed and introduced into eggs which, in turn, were placed under the bird. These arrangements were crude, but they served their purpose.

His discovery of lung fluke, *Paragonimus westermani*, illustrates how a trained observer can recognize the importance of the most unexpected incidents. Although this fluke had been found in 1878 in the lungs of a tiger in a European zoo, Manson was the first to isolate it in humans and label it the cause of endemic hemoptysis:

> I was not looking for this parasite when I found it, for a man may search for a shilling and find a sovereign. The important thing is to search. . . . On one occasion a petty Chinese mandarin came for consultation about an eruption on his hands which proved to be itch. During the examination he coughed and ejected the sputum on the floor of my consulting room. My disgust and anger at such an exhibition of bad manners evaporated on seeing the sputum was tinged with blood. "Here," I thought, "is another opportunity," so instead of reproaching him for spitting on my carpet, requested him to repeat the cough and this time to deposit the sputum in a watchglass. He very obligingly did so. My forbearance was rewarded. On placing a little of the rusty sputum under the microscope I found it to be loaded with little brown operculated bodies, manifestly the ova of a parasite, to me quite a new one.

A number of other notable discoveries were made while in the Far East or after Manson's return to London. These included descriptions of *Sparganum mansoni*, the larval stage of *Filaria loa*, the eggs of *Schistosoma mansoni*, *Trypanosoma gambiense*, and the fungus *Trichophyton mansoni*, as well as clinical descriptions of tinea imbricata and tropical sprue.

In 1883 Manson left Amoy for Hong Kong because his growing family demanded a larger income. He often looked back "with great pleasure to my residence in Amoy. . . . The Chinese hospital was the principal source of interest to me, where, on several days of the week, I spent my forenoon and on Saturday, the afternoon operating and investigating. It was my laboratory, my school. There I gained whatever experience and knowledge I may possess of tropical medicine." He practiced medicine in Hong Kong for 6 years. His greatest accomplishments during this time were in medical education. He founded the Hongkong Medical Society, of which he became the first president. He initiated medical teaching at the Alice

Memorial Hospital and was one of the prime movers in the foundation of the Hongkong Medical College in 1887, as well as its first dean. Sun Yat-sen was in the initial class of this school. Sir James Cantile, one of the other founders of the Hongkong Medical College, described him in this way:

> The first student to join the classes was Sun Yat-sen. Of some twenty-four men who presented themselves, I was most attracted by Sun. Himself a Christian and the son of a Christian, he at once arrested my attention by his gentleness of character, his earnestness in study, and by his behavior as a gentleman in the College and in private life. He was the model and the example to the other members of the classes, and then, as throughout his whole career, he attracted by his personality both teachers and fellow-students.

In 1889 Manson returned to his native Scotland. His years of hard work in China had been profitable, and he had put away enough money to retire, or so he thought. Within a year, owing to both family misfortunes and depreciation of the Hong Kong dollar, he was forced to return to work. To facilitate this, he moved to London to begin practice as a consultant. Manson's reputation had been unequaled in the East, and patients had sought him out. The situation in London was different. There were many excellent surgeons, and his expertise in tropical diseases was not needed. He soon discovered that it was not easy to start a new practice at the age of 46. It was not long, however, before he was appointed a physician to the Seaman's Hospital Society, in charge of a number of beds in the Dreadnought Hospital at Greenwich. There he found a mass of unutilized clinical material that was of great interest to him, and soon he was on familiar ground. Patients with diseases of which he had unique knowledge and experience were common. He was once again the sought-after consultant. He quickly observed that beriberi was prevalent among seamen who flocked to the port of London from various tropical regions. The various parasitic diseases he had learned about in the Orient abounded. He was soon giving demonstrations and lectures on these disorders. Furthermore, he was able to continue his research, and he soon confirmed and extended the recent discoveries regarding the malaria parasite. Other parasitic diseases that he had not previously investigated now drew his attention. Many cases of guineaworm infection came under his care, and he was able to demonstrate the remarkable life history of this parasite and trace its development in the body cavity of a species of cyclops that he captured in a pond at Hampstead Heath. His studies were not limited to patients directly under his care. Friends sent him blood slides from all parts of the world. Using these, as well as fresh specimens from patients who came to him from far-off exotic locales, he was able in a short time to describe, for the first time, three new species of blood filariae.

In a small room at the top of his house, referred to as "the muck room," he carried out experiments on mice, rats, and birds. He even artificially bred various species of mosquito. This humble room soon became the meeting ground for all those in London who were interested in the development of this new branch of science that was to become known as tropical medicine.

About 1897, Manson initiated a series of lectures on tropical diseases, hoping that this would stimulate the British government to provide special instruction on the entire range of tropical medicine. This idea was neither far-fetched nor impractical. The British Empire was in its heyday and had extensive involvement in tropical regions. Service in the tropical British colonies was associated with extremely high mortality. If the teaching of tropical medicine could help cut down this terrible toll, the British colonial administration and the economic life of Great Britain itself would benefit, to say nothing of the saving of lives and health of those working in the tropics. In this effort Manson found a firm supporter in Joseph Chamberlain, to many historians the greatest colonial secretary Great Britain ever had. With Chamberlain's support, Manson's plan was adopted. In 1899 the London School of Tropical Medicine opened at the Albert Dock. Manson taught there almost daily, and soon he came to be regarded as the oracle of tropical medicine, and beyond that as the personal guide and friend of every student who entered the school. The London School of Tropical Medicine later became part of the famous London School of Hygiene and Tropical Medicine.

Manson's other accomplishments during his London years, including the founding of the Royal Society of Tropical Medicine, were numerous, as were the honors he received.

One of his interests was the role of mosquitoes in the transmission of malaria. The first great step in the battle against malaria was taken in 1880 by Charles Louis Alphonse Laveran, who discovered the causative organism. Laveran was a French army surgeon who was serving in Algeria. Working much as Manson had in China, with simple, even primitive, equipment, he was able to find the microscopic parasite of malaria in the blood of patients suffering from the disease. He published a total of four papers on malaria and in 1907 received a Nobel prize for his work. He observed the various stages through which the parasite passed and noted that with each new invasion of parasites into the bloodstream there was a bout of fever. Laveran's discoveries, important as they were, did not answer the question of how malaria could be controlled. In order to do this, the mode of transmission of the parasite had to be known. Only the added information that the mosquito spread the parasite would transform Laveran's observations into a practical advance. It was in the study of this crucial step that Manson played a role.

Manson was still in China when Laveran made his discovery. He did not even hear of it until 5 years later. He then tried to confirm Laveran's work. He looked for the parasite in the blood of patients, but during the time he was in China he could not find it. He finally succeeded in doing so in London in 1892. Seeing the malaria parasite itself increased his interest in malaria. It was clear to him that the parasite must have an intermediate host and that the host must play the pivotal role in spreading the disease. His knowledge of filariae led him to suggest that this host was the mosquito. He stated this hypothesis in a paper, "On the Nature and Significance of the Crescentic and Flagellated Bodies in Malarial Blood," that appeared December 8, 1894, in the *British Medical Journal*:

> The Mosquito having been shown to be the agent by which the filaria is removed from the human blood-vessels, this or a similar suctorial insect must be the agent which removes from the human blood-vessels those forms of the malarial organism which are destined to continue the existence of this organism outside the body. It must, therefore, be in this or a similar suctorial insect or insects that the first stages of the extra-corporeal life of the malarial organism are passed.

It was not Manson, but Sir Ronald Ross, who established the life cycle of the malaria parasite and won a Nobel prize. In 1889, Ross came to London from India, where he had been serving as a surgeon in the Indian medical service. He came to London to study bacteriology and became a diplomat in public health. It was while he was studying in London that he met Manson. Manson showed Ross the malaria parasite in human blood and expressed the opinion that what they were seeing probably represented only a single phase of a more elaborate life cycle. He advised Ross to pursue this avenue of research and suggested to Ross that malaria, like filariasis, was probably spread by mosquitoes. Ross was already aware that Laveran had made the same suggestion, but he nonetheless "was tremendously impressed with the argument and determined to test the hypothesis thoroughly on my return to India." Whether or not Ross would have studied the subject if this conversation had not taken place is impossible to tell. But the work that proved that mosquitoes spread malaria was done by Ross alone. It was Ross who discovered the complete life history of the malarial parasite. During the 4 years he spent on this investigation, Ross wrote 110 letters to Manson in which he described his progress. Manson, on his part, was not merely a passive observer. He kept up his end of the correspondence with encouragement and advice. He also made sure that others interested in Ross's work were kept informed. He examined the numerous specimens that Ross sent him and wrote strong letters to government officials in England urging them to do all they could to help Ross carry on his research. He personally saw Lord Lister and Joseph Chamberlain and implored them to get the authorities to give Ross the facilities he needed. He even got Lord Lister to come to his house to see the slides Ross had sent him, and he persuaded the Royal Society to send Dr. Daniels to India to help Ross.

Ross's working conditions in India were not much different than Manson's had been in Amoy. He worked with a dilapidated microscope in a makeshift laboratory with equipment that would be considered extremely primitive by present-day standards.

Ross's efforts finally met with success in 1897, when at Secunderabad he discovered the malaria parasite in the stomach of an Anopheles mosquito that had been fed on a patient with malaria named Husein Khan. This was the pivotal step, reminiscent of Manson's revolutionary discovery in his study of *Filaria*. Ross then went beyond Manson, who had never traced the development of the parasite in the intermediate host nor shown that the host actively spread the disease by biting another human. Ross traced the development of the *Plasmodium* in the mosquito, finding the zygote, or sexual forms, in the stomach and the sporoblasts, or progeny, in the salivary glands. In the summer of 1898 Ross furnished the final proof that the mosquito was the intermediary host for malaria and actually spread the disease when he infected healthy birds by the bites of mosquitoes that had previously bitten birds known to have malaria.

This discovery fired Manson's enthusiasm. It was a key discovery that needed to be known and appreciated throughout the world. In order to make the general public aware of the importance of the part played by the mosquito in malaria, Manson obtained some live mosquitoes carrying malaria from the malarial marshes near Rome. These mosquitoes were then allowed to bite two healthy Londoners, one of whom was his own son. Both, of course, got malaria, and the malaria parasites were recovered from their blood. He also arranged for two English doctors to live in a malaria-plagued marsh at the mouth of the Tiber for 14 weeks at the height of the malarial season. They went out and around during the day, but for the whole period they remained in a mosquito-proof hut from an hour before sunset to an hour after sunrise. Because the malarial mosquito bites only at night, these two physicians did not get malaria, whereas the unprotected people around them suffered severely from the disease.

Always a poet, Ross expressed his elation at his scientific victory in verse:

> This day designing God
>   Hath put into my hand
> A wondrous thing. And God
>   Be praised. At His command,
> I have found thy secret deeds
>   One million-murdering Death.
> I know that this little thing
>   A million men will save—
> Oh death where is thy sting?
>   Thy victory oh grave?

In more prosaic terms, Ross wrote of his discovery as follows:

> The exact route of infection of this great disease which annually slays its millions of human beings and keeps whole continents in darkness was revealed. These minute spores enter the salivary glands of the mosquito, and pass with its poisonous saliva directly into the blood of men. Never in our dreams had we imagined so wonderful a tale as this.

Ross retired from the Indian medical service in 1899. He was then appointed lecturer on tropical medicine at the University of Liverpool. He was awarded the Nobel prize in medicine in 1902, and he became Sir Ronald Ross in 1911 when he was knighted.

While Manson and Ross were safely in London and India pursuing parasites, Sun Yat-sen had given up medicine for the more precarious life of a political activist. Sun Yat-sen's father was a convert to Christianity and was employed as a missionary agent by the London Missionary Society. Because of these connections, at the age of 18 Sun was able to obtain employment in the hospital of the Anglo-American mission in Canton. There he became deeply interested in medicine, and in 1886, at the age of 20, he joined the newly organized college of medicine in Hong Kong.

He was a brilliant student, as borne out by the fact that in his first 2 years of study he gained several scholastic distinctions. He was first in chemistry, minor surgery, and clinical observation, and second in botany, physics, and physiology, and he received the prestigious Watson scholarship. Of the seven who had started in the first class of the college in 1886, two completed the curriculum in 1892, and Sun Yat-sen was one of these two successful students.

After graduation, Sun settled in the Portuguese colony of Macao and opened a private practice. He was influenced in this choice, no doubt, by the fact that Macao was near the village where he had been born and therefore was in a district in which he had many friends and relatives. These, he hoped, would help overcome the continuing resistance of most Chinese to Western medicine, at least as practiced by him. Macao had a large and well-built hospital, but the treatment was by traditional Chinese methods. He impressed on the governors of the hospital the benefits of Western medicine, and the latter agreed to devote one wing of the hospital to the practice of Western medicine under Sun Yat-sen. His old professor, Dr. James Cantile, was most supportive: "I encouraged him especially in surgical work. When major operations had to be done, I went on several occasions to Macao to assist him, and there, in the presence of the governors of the hospital, he performed important operations."

From Macao, Sun later moved to Manson's old stamping ground, Amoy. There he was nominally engaged in the practice of medicine, but he was actively organizing an "association for the regeneration of China." In 1895 an attempt by these reformers to capture Canton failed, and Sun barely escaped with his life back to Macao.

There was then a price on his head, and China and the various colonial outposts such as Macao and Hong Kong could no longer be regarded as safe for him. Sun fled to London, where he was warmly greeted by his old teachers Cantile and Manson. A few days later, when he was walking near the Chinese legation in Portland Place, two Chinese approached him, enticed him into the legation, and, acting under orders from Peking, kept him prisoner. With the help of one of the English servants in the legation, Sun managed to get a note to Manson. After communicating with the police and the Foreign Office, Manson called at the Chinese legation and demanded to see Sun Yat-sen. The attendant denied that he was there. Manson, however, discovered that Sun was to be smuggled down to the docks that night and taken to China. He and Cantile remained in a cab outside the legation all night in order to prevent Sun Yat-sen's removal. On the next day, reinforcements arrived in the person of the Foreign Office representative, who demanded Sun Yat-sen's release, a demand that was quickly met, because that was still the day of gunboat diplomacy, when empires were still empires.

China continued, of course, to smolder with demands for political change and Sun Yat-sen soon returned to the fray. In 1908 the aged dowager empress died, leaving the government in the hands of a weak regency for the 3-year-old prince. This regency fell in 1911, and on February 12, 1912, a republic was proclaimed, with Dr. Sun Yat-sen as provisional president. But the support of the republic was unstable, and Sun resigned in favor of Yuan Shih-kai, who had been an able general and aide to the dowager empress and had much better support, especially in the north. Sun and the Nationalist or Kuomintang party, which he had organized, remained suspicious of this remnant of the old monarchy. When Yuan Shih-kai began to usurp power, the Kuomintang revolted (1913). Yuan crushed the revolt and became military dictator of part of China, but overall the political situations in China remained in turmoil because of the power struggles of various local warlords and the economic and political domination of various sectors by foreign powers, especially Japan and Russia. Throughout it all, Sun Yat-sen stood for a unified republic, but although the Kuomintang had set up a separate government in Canton, there was still a national government in Peking, and warlords controlled many provinces. Sun Yat-sen and the Kuomintang made little headway in uniting the country, and in 1925 Sun went to Peking to confer with two warlords and died.

Sun's death set the stage for the next acts in China's tragedy. Not long before his death, Sun had invited Soviet advisers to China. The Russians taught the Nationalist army officers modern war techniques. Sun apparently had become disenchanted with the Soviets prior to his death, but not so his wife, who after Sun's death became a leader in the Communist movement in China.

Chiang Kai-shek, who was commander of the Kuomintang army, assumed power once Sun was out of the way and moved on to Peking, which he finally captured in 1929. By this time the Nationalist government controlled the entire country, at least nominally. However, the Kuomintang party had split down the middle, with one section becoming ardent Communists and the other, led by Chiang, staunchly anti-Communist. This breach soon became a protracted war that continued on the Chinese mainland until the final Communist victory in 1949. Such was the political life and legacy of the man whose life was once saved by the founder of tropical medicine.

NOTES

The most complete biography of Sir Patrick Manson is P. H. Manson-Bahr's *The Life and Work of Sir Patrick Manson* (London: Cassel and Co., 1927). Of the numerous shorter sketches of his life, the two I like best are found in collections of biographies: Sir William Hale White's *Great Doctors of the Nineteenth Century* (London: Edward Arnold and Co.) also has a sketch of Sir Ronald Ross. M. E. M. Walker's *Pioneers of Public Health* (Freeport, N.Y.: Books for Libraries Press) also includes studies of Alphonse Laveran and Sir Ronald Ross.

Many of Manson's original writings are included in the two-volume set *Tropical Medicine and Parasitology*, edited by B. H. Kean, K. E. Mott, and A. J. Russell (Ithaca: Cornell University Press).

Francesco Redi
and
The Discovery of Spectacles

Much has been written, ranging from the valuable to the worthless, about the invention of eyeglasses; but when it is all summed up, the fact remains that the world has found lenses on its nose without knowing whom to thank.

Vasco Ronchi (1946)

If Redi had done nothing else than help to preserve this priceless mirror of the late Renaissance, he would have earned, by that alone, the undying gratitude of posterity.

Rufus Cole (1926) discussing Redi's copy of the original manuscript of Benvenuto Cellini's autobiography

Francesco Redi and
The Discovery of Spectacles

The first extensive discussion of the invention of eyeglasses was written by Francesco Redi (1626–1697), a well-known seventeenth-century physician, naturalist, and poet. According to his account, the person most responsible for the invention of eyeglasses was Friar Alessandro Spina, a monk from the Dominican monastery of St. Catherine of Pisa. Redi's friend Carlo Roberto Dati was also interested in tracing the history of spectacles, and in 1673, Redi, having heard of Dati's interest, related some of his views on the subject in a letter:

> Friar Alessandro Spina of Pisa made with his own hands whatever he wished, and shared it with others, since he was dominated by kindness. At that time, through a beautiful, useful and novel invention, somebody invented the glass lenses which are commonly called "eye-glasses" and did not want to communicate to anybody the art of making them. Having seen them, this good man, a craftsman, mastered them immediately without anybody teaching him, and he taught others who wanted to know. He sang melodiously, wrote elegantly and decorated the handwritten books which are called illuminated manuscripts. In short, there was none of the manual arts that he did not know.

According to Redi and Dati, who derived his data from Redi, Spina was at least a partial discoverer of eyeglasses, who having merely seen or heard of eyeglasses was able to discover how to manufacture them himself. This was a remarkable accomplishment, similar to Galileo's role in developing the telescope, an analogy that was certainly not lost on Redi. Redi later wrote that if Friar Alessandro Spina was not the first inventor of eyeglasses, at least this beloved monk, by himself, without any instruction, rediscovered the method of making eyeglasses. Furthermore, it was through Spina's willingness to share his discovery that this most useful invention was actually made available. Redi was quick to point out that virtually the same thing had happened "by a certain coincidence of fate, to our most famous Galileo Galilei. Having heard the report that a certain Fleming had invented the long spyglass, which is called by the Greek name telescope; he worked out a similar one solely with the aid of the theory of refractions, without even having seen that which the Fleming had invented."

Redi thus pictured Spina as the one man most responsible for giving the gift of corrective lenses to mankind. But the truth is far from Redi's retelling of it. Spina's role was not that of discoverer or even rediscoverer. He had not simply heard of the concept of eyeglasses and then divined how to produce them; he had actually seen them in use, and after seeing and examining them, he was able to reproduce them and pass this skill on to others. He was neither a discoverer nor rediscoverer, merely a copier who today would be liable to legal action for having infringed on someone else's patent. Why did Redi attempt to attribute to Spina such a major role? Why was his attempt so successful? The second of these questions is easier to answer. Redi's version was believed, and in many circles still is believed, because it was written by Redi, and Francesco Redi was one of the greatest writer-scientists of his age or any age.

Redi was born in 1626 in Arezzo which was the ancestral seat of the Redi family, long prominent in Tuscan affairs. His father was physician to the Grand Duke of Tuscany, and much of Francesco's boyhood was spent in Florence. At that time, Florence was perhaps the most interesting city in Europe and a most suitable locale for the appearance of a true artist-scientist. By the beginning of the seventeenth century, Dante and Petrarch, Ghiberti and Donatello, Michelangelo, Raphael, Fra Angelico, Botticelli, Leonardo da Vinci, and Benvenuto Cellini, whose names had been linked with Florence in an earlier age, were all long dead and buried. But their works were still to be found throughout the city. If today one cannot visit Florence without feeling the influence of these masters who once walked the same streets and worked and created such beauty there, how much more profound their influence must have been on a brilliant Tuscan youth 3 centuries ago, when it was still possible to contemplate their accomplishments undisturbed by the sounds and smells of Vespas.

Florence reached its zenith by the end of the fifteenth century. Its decline began with the end of the older branch of the Medici family. It cannot be denied that the art and learning of Florence no longer had the same brilliance under the younger branch of the Medici family. Nevertheless, during the seventeenth century, science, that late bloomer of the Renaissance, began to blossom in Florence, with far-reaching and significant results. It was during the height of this golden age of science that Francesco Redi lived and worked in Florence. The previous 100 years had witnessed a number of events that helped nurture the development of science in Florence. The most important of these helped to decrease reliance on authority as the absolute arbiter of scientific truth.

For the first time in 14 centuries, man had resumed the study of his own anatomic structure directly with his own eyes. Instead of reliance on ancient medical authors and reverence for ancient descriptions, dissection and direct observation began to become recognized as the superior means. In 1543 this break with tradition had been signaled by the publication of Vesalius's masterpiece. Such innovation was not limited to the study of anatomy. In astronomy, Copernicus and Kepler had given man's mind an entirely new conception of the universe, a solar system of which the sun, not the earth, was the center. This scientific discovery based on direct observation challenged the two great sources of authority: the ancients and the church.

Most important for Francesco Redi was the fact that at the time of his birth there lived in Florence one great and lonely man who was investigating nature with the new tools and new methods of the day. When Redi was 6 years old, this man, Galileo, was brought to Rome by the Inquisition. Following his trial he was allowed to live in the seclusion of his villa near Florence. Seclusion from the world was the prescribed condition of Galileo's comparative freedom. He died in 1642, when Francesco was 16 years old. Although Redi's later scientific studies were not concerned with the problems on which Galileo had worked, Redi's approach to science and his reliance on observation rather than authority owe much to Galileo's influence. Those who are disturbed by the slow pace that typifies the American judicial system may take heart in the news that the trial of Galileo has now been officially reopened for review.

After completing his studies in a Jesuit school, Redi entered the University of Pisa, and in 1647 he received the combined degree of doctor of medicine and philosophy, not an unusual procedure in those days. At that time the leading universities of Italy were Padua, Bologna, and Pisa. Padua, which was under the control of Venice, was the chief rival of the University of Pisa, which was under the direct protection of the Grand Duke of Tuscany. It was from Padua that Galileo had been persuaded to come to Florence as mathematician and philosopher to the Grand Duke.

After graduation, Redi spent some 5 years traveling through Europe to extend and complete his education. During his years of travel he seems to have spent much time in Rome, working in the Vatican libraries and indulging his tastes as a bibliophile and collector of manuscripts. To his interest and discrimination in collecting manuscripts we owe one of our greatest literary possessions, for the manuscript of Benvenuto Cellini's autobiography was preserved in Redi's collection. At the age of 26, he returned to Florence and began to practice medicine. His father was at that time the personal physician to the Grand Duke, a position to which Francesco succeeded at age 40. Redi apparently was a wise and skillful physician, and this, combined with his charm and versatility, made him much in demand among the wealthy and powerful. In his treatments he demonstrated a skepticism that was somewhat unusual for the time, and it is said he told his patients that there was one thing to be feared more than the diseases from which they suffered, namely, the medicines that were offered to cure them. He returned to Hippocratic simplicity in treatment and was a great advocate of the use of water. His contributions to clinical medicine are preserved in his "Consultations." These are the records of about 100 cases in which description, treatment, and prognosis are presented. However, his medical work does not show extraordinary brilliance, nor does it appear that he was greatly interested in the purely clinical features of disease. His greatest work lay in other directions, in the study of certain fundamental biological problems and in parasitology, and it is because of his discoveries in these fields that he still deserves our attention.

Redi's first important independent scientific work, "Ossevazione intorno alle Vipere," was written in 1664. In this paper Redi described the studies he had made with various poisonous serpents, describing the poison glands and the fangs from which the poison is injected. He described his own experiments that demonstrated for the first time that snake venom must be injected under the skin to produce its effect and that when such venoms are introduced into the stomach with food they are harmless.

To us, it seems obvious that snake venoms are poisonous only when injected, not when swallowed. This was not always so widely known. In fact, 50 years after the publication of Redi's study on vipers, the two greatest living Italian physicians debated this issue in regard to the death of Cleopatra (see Addendum 1).

In 1668 Redi published another work: *Experiments Concerning Diverse Natural Objects and Especially Those which Are Brought from India*. This book was written in the form of a long letter to Padre Atanasio Circher, who was head of the Jesuit College in Rome, and it was written to refute the extravagant and marvelous medical claims made by Jesuit missionaries in India and America. Redi took great pains to disprove the popular belief in the efficacy of so-called serpent stones in curing snakebite. He showed by repeated experiments on animals that this form of treatment was entirely without beneficial effect. In some respects this work by Redi resembles the *Pseudodoxia* of Sir Thomas Browne that had been published a short time before (1645). However, rather than refuting error with error (or, at any rate, with opinions that seemed more reasonable than the original ones), as did Browne, Redi overthrew popular misconceptions by sound evidence, often gathered in experiments he himself had performed.

Redi's most significant work, the one that has done the most to maintain his reputation as a scientist, was his *Esperienze intorno alla Generazioni dege Insetti* (*Experiments Concerning the Generation of Insects*). This was published in 1668, and within 20 years five editions had appeared. In his introduction, Redi reviewed the current beliefs:

> After a long period of fertility, during which time many monstrous and marvelous generations were brought forth, the Earth Mother became at last exhausted and sterile and lost her power of producing man and the larger animals, still she retained enough vigor to bring forth (besides plants, that are presumed to be generated spontaneously) certain small creatures, such as flies, wasps, spiders, ants, scorpions and all other terrestrial and aerial insects. The schools both ancient and modern all agree in this, and constantly teach that the Earth has continued to produce these creatures and will produce them as long as she exists. They do not, however, agree as to the manner in which these insects are generated, nor how life is communicated to them; for they say that not only does the Earth possess this occult power, but that it is possessed, by all animals, living and dead, also by all things produced from the Earth, and finally by those which are about to decay and return to dust. Hence others have claimed putrefaction itself to be the all-potent cause of generation, and still others, natural heat.

In the seventeenth century, virtually everyone believed that if the conditions were right the rod of Aaron was not needed to bring forth a plague of frogs or locusts. Even that great rebel Paracelsus had been a strong proponent of spontaneous generation.

Redi also gave an interesting account of the origin of the view that bees are born in the decayed flesh of bulls, tracing it to statements of the early Greek writers. Antigonus Carystius had written that in order to breed bees, a whole bullock must be buried underground, with only the horns protruding. In due time, if these are sawed off, bees swarm out. Redi also quoted Thomas Monfet, who wrote that some bees are born in the flesh of bullocks but others are born in the flesh of lions, and the latter are better, stronger, and more courageous. The lion fable probably originated from the biblical story of Samson, who, on the first of his several romantic liaisons, killed a young lion. Later, on returning for another visit, he saw that the carcass was filled with bees and honey.

Redi rejected the authority of current opinion on this problem, despite its support by both Aristotle and the Bible, a stand that can only be viewed as courageous, especially because he had been so close to the experience of Galileo. However, Redi expressed his strong disbelief that bees generated spontaneously in the carcasses of either bullocks or lions. Because outright disagreement with the Bible could have caused him a great deal of trouble, even though he might safely differ with Aristotle, Redi logically explained away the story of Samson and the bees. Redi conceded that bees did appear in the lion's carcass, as Samson observed, but that this observation did not warrant the conclusion that the bees were generated there. The sacred text does not state that the bees were given birth within the lion's putrefying body. The Hebrew text says only that Samson returned after "some days" and saw the bees and their honey. Redi believed that there was enough evidence to suggest that "some days" really meant a long delay of a year. After a delay of this long, Redi believed, it was probable that nothing was left but a bony skeleton, inside of which the bees might well have collected and gone about their business of making honey.

Redi's book contains not only arguments such as these and poetic quotations but also experimental evidence. The gist of his experimental study was as follows: Redi killed three snakes and placed them in an open box, allowing them to decay. Not long afterward, he noted that the snakes were covered with cone-shaped worms, apparently legless (maggots). After the maggots had consumed all the meat, they disappeared. To discover what had become of them, he repeated the experiment, but this time, when the meat was all consumed, he covered every exit from the box. On the 19th day, some of the worms became quiet, appeared to shrink, and gradually assumed an egglike shape. He noticed that there were some differences in the appearances of these eggs (which we now call pupae), and he segregated them in glass vessels covered with paper. At the end of 8 days, the shells of the eggs in one vessel were broken, and each pupae gave rise to a green fly. A second variety of pupae were placed in a second vessel, and on the 14th day appeared large black flies. From the pupae of another kind came black flies striped with white. Redi then took various kinds of dead animals: pigeon, capon, pieces of veal, sheep's heart, raw and cooked flesh of ox, deer, buffalo, lion, tiger, and so forth and repeated the experiment. In every case the result was the same, and one or the other kind of fly developed, sometimes all kinds. As he continued these studies, he observed that besides the flies and the worms the meat was also covered with the eggs from which the worms were hatched. "Having considered these things, I began to believe that all worms found in meat were derived directly from the droppings of flies, and not from the putrefaction of the meat," especially because "before the meat became covered with worms, flies had hovered over it: Flies of the same kind as those which later were bred in the meat." But, he said, "belief would be vain without the confirmation of experiment, hence in the middle of July

I put a snake, some fish, some eels of the Arno, and a slice of milk-fed veal in four large, wide-mouth flasks: Having well covered and sealed them, I then filled the same number of flasks in the same way, only leaving these open." He went on to tell that in the closed flasks no worms developed, even after many days, whereas in the open flasks flies were seen entering and leaving at will, and the meat became worm-infested. These and similar experiments were repeated time and time again. He reported the following:

> Although I thought I had proved that flesh of dead animals could not engender worms unless the semina of live ones were deposited therein, still to remove all doubt, as the trial had been made with closed vessels into which the air could not penetrate or circulate, I wished to attempt a new experiment by putting meat and fish in a large vessel closed only with a fine Naples veil, that allowed the air to enter. For a further protection against flies, I placed the vessel in a frame covered with the same net. No worms ever developed in the meat, though many flies buzzed about and lighted on the outside of the net and deposited eggs there.

It is not necessary to remark on the great similarity between this crucial experiment and those performed over 200 years later by Pasteur in order to finally settle the problem of spontaneous generation of microorganisms. It is self-evident that Redi could not discuss spontaneous generation of bacteria and other microorganisms, because their existence at that time was not even suspected. However, Redi did extend his experiments to include bees, scorpions, spiders, and the worms that were popularly and erroneously believed to arise spontaneously in vegetables and decayed fruits, as well as dead wood and live trees. Redi finally stated the following:

> Although content to be corrected by any one wiser than myself, if I should make erroneous statements, I shall express my belief that the Earth, after having brought forth the first plants and animals at the beginning by order of the Supreme and Omnipotent Creator, has never since produced any kind of plants or animals, either perfect or imperfect; and everything which we know in past or present time she has produced, came solely from true seeds of the plants and animals themselves, which thus, through means of their own, preserve their species.

Although Redi may not have been the first to express an opinion opposed to the idea of spontaneous generation, he was undoubtedly the first to use experimental evidence to justify his beliefs. Redi's later scientific work consisted largely in investigations of animal parasites, studies probably stimulated by his interest in spontaneous generation. His *Osservazioni intorno agli animali viventi che si trovano negli animali viventi* appeared in 1684, and in it Redi described 108 different species, including cestodes, trematodes, nematodes, acanthocephales, acarines, and insects, that were isolated from a great variety of animals, including the hare, dog, wolf, cat, various fish, lion, tiger, and man. If a rare animal was captured or died in the menagerie, Redi was at once notified, and he made a careful search for parasites. In his work on pediculi he stated that he was unable to discover any pediculi on lions and tigers, but "the search for parasites on these animals is attended with considerable difficulty."

The most important aspect of this work probably was his demonstration of the reproductive organs in the ascaris of man and his demonstration of ascaris eggs.

Such discoveries must have gone far in dispelling his remaining doubts about the impossibility of spontaneous generation, and they helped assure his place as the father of the science of parasitology. Although among physicians and scientists Redi is best known for his work regarding spontaneous generation, he lives in the hearts of his countrymen as a poet. It cannot be claimed that he ranks as a great Italian poet, but his poetry is not without merit and is still read. The one poem for which he is best remembered is in praise of the various vintages of Tuscan wine. Entitled "Bacco in Tuscany," it was published in 1685 and translated into English in 1825 by Leigh Hunt.

Bacchus in Tuscany

The conqueror of the East, the God of Wine,
Taking his rounds divine,
Pitch'd his blith sojourn on the Tuscan hills;
And where the imperial seat
First feels the morning heat,
Lo, on the lawn, with May-time white and red,
He sat with Ariadne on a day,
And as he stand, and as he quaff'd away,
He kiss'd his charmer first, and thus said:—
   Dearest, if one's vital tide
Ran not with the grape's beside,
What would life be, (short of Cupid?)
Much too short, and far too stupid.
You see the beam here from the sky
That tips the goblet in mine eye:
Vines are nets that catch such food,
And then turn them into sparkling blood.
Come then—in the beverage bold
Let's renew us and grow muscular;
And for those who're getting old,
Glasses get of size majuscular;
And dancing and in feasting,
Quips, and cranks, and worlds of jesting,
Let us, with a laughing eye,
See the old boy Time go by,
Who with his eternal sums
Whirls his brains and wastes his thumbs.
Away with thinking! miles with care!
Hallo, you knaves! the goblets there.

Although the poem is too long to be repeated entirely, his lines on Chianti are worth noting:

True son of the earth Chianti wine,
Born on the ground of a gypsy vine;
Born on the ground for sturdy souls,
And not the rank race of one of your poles.
   Like a king,
In his conquering,
Chianti wine with his red flag goes

Down to my heart, and down to my toes:
He makes no noise, he beats no drums;
Yet pain and trouble fly as he comes.

Redi usually is placed among the Arcadians, a group of poets who collected in Italy around the expatriate Queen Christina of Sweden. This remarkable woman was a daughter of Gustavus Adolphus. She renounced her throne to live in Italy and act as a patron of letters and science. A collection of 60 of Redi's sonnets was published in 1703.

During his life, Redi became a member of all of the notable literary societies of Italy, and before his death he was elected arch-counsel of the Accademia della Crusca, the highest office in the most illustrious of such groups. His last years, however, were not happy, for he was bothered by recurrent attacks that his biographers all refer to as epilepsy. The exact nature of these attacks in not entirely clear, and they may well have been angina pectoris. Chiefly as a direct outgrowth of the fame of his poem in praise of wine, Redi, through the years, acquired a reputation as an epicure and profligate. Although he was not entirely lacking in appreciation of earthly joys, it seems that Redi, at least in his later life, was temperate if not absolutely abstemious. Redi was never married, but late in life he became the mainstay of his entire family. His brothers, it seems, accomplished little with their lives, other than trouble for Francesco. One of his brothers was married and had a family, but Redi actually supported the family and eventually adopted the children. In spite of his illness, Redi kept on working, though apparently constantly in fear of an attack. His fear was justified, for as a result of one of his attacks, he died suddenly one night at Pisa. His body was carried to Arezzo and placed in the church of San Francesco. A suitable tomb was later erected by his nephew and adopted heir, Gregoire. On the tomb are these simple words: "Francisco Redio Patricio Aretino Gregoriis Fratris Filius," as if to indicate that his name was so glorious that posterity would need no eulogy.

Today, a statue of Redi can be found in the Uffizi Gallery in Florence. It is most appropriate that this statue of Redi should stand there, for it is to Redi that we owe the wonderful Uffizi collection of marbles. The story is told that Cosimo Medici, who frequently was encumbered by overeating and excessive drinking, was advised by Redi to take regular walks. Cosimo decided to follow this advice by walking regularly in the great corridor of the Uffizi, and to amuse himself during this time of exercise he decided to assemble there all the marbles belonging to the Medici family. He thus collected there all the wonderful statues that until then had been scattered about, many as far away as the Villa Medici in Rome.

Why, then, did this great and respected man of such depth and breadth exaggerate the role of Spina in the invention of eyeglasses? The exact reason is unknown. He enjoyed practical jokes, but that alone is not a sufficient explanation. Redi was fiercely patriotic. He loved Tuscany and perhaps wanted to embellish its glory. Certainly many others have claimed inventions for their native lands for this reason. Furthermore, by analogy, his glorification of Spina's role might reflect increased honor on his hero Galileo, who did for the telescope what Spina did for eyeglasses. But if Spina was not the inventor, who was?

Friar Giordano da Rivalto, an eloquent preacher of the order of Saint Dominic, gave a sermon on February 23, 1306, in the church of Santa Maria Novella in Florence in which he made the following remarks:

> It is not yet twenty years since there was found the art of making eyeglasses which make for good vision, one of the best arts and most necessary that the world has. . . . So short a time it is since there was invented a new art that never existed. I have seen the man who first invented and created it and I have talked to him.

Who was this great benefactor of mankind to whom Friar Giordano talked? Certainly not the copier Spina. Had it been Spina, Giordano would certainly have mentioned his name, because Spina was a fellow Dominican, and thus naming him would have brought fame to the order, and Friar Giordano never missed an opportunity to do that. Furthermore, had it been Spina, the remark "I have seen the man . . . and I have talked to him" would have been unnecessary. In place of Spina, another Tuscan has been suggested, none other than Salvino degli Armati. In 1684, some 6 years after Redi's version of the discovery of eyeglasses was written, Ferdinando Leopoldo del Migliore published a historical guide to his native Florence. In his description of the church of Santa Maria Maggiore, the chapels of which had been renovated just shortly before his birth, del Migliore wrote the following:

> There was another memorial which went to ruin in the restoration of that church. It is faithfully recorded, however, in our ancient register of burials. It is very precious because by means of it we came to know about the first inventor of eyeglasses. He was a gentleman of this country! Florence, which is so highly renowned for genius in every subject requiring keenness of mind. He was Messer Salvino degl' Armati, son of Armato, of a noble family which continues to give its name today to Chiasso degl' Armati, that short alley (for that is what "chiasso" means) situated behind the Centaur. The statue of this man in ordinary dress was to be seen reclining on a large slab with letters around it, which said the following:

> *Here lies Salvino degli Armati, son of Armato, of Florence, inventor of eye-glasses. May God forgive his sins. A.D. 1317.*

> He is the one who is not named or specified by the ancient manuscript Chronicle in the monastery of the Dominican Fathers of Pisa. Francesco Redi, a most excellent doctor of our times, quoted this Chronicle in his learned report on eyeglasses. In it we read that Friar Alessandro Spina, who lived in those same times and who perhaps was a Florentine and not a Pisan, sought to learn about the invention of making eyeglasses from someone who knew it and did not want to divulge it, and that by himself Spina found a way of making them.

So now we know the true discoverer of spectacles. But can we be sure?

Del Migliore's version was certainly quickly accepted and seconded by Manni, who wrote an entire book, *Historical Treatise about Eyeglasses, Invented by Salvino Armati, a Florentine Gentleman*, that won widespread acceptance of del Migliore's candidate for the role of inventor of eyeglasses.

The reclining statue of Salvino with its accompanying epitaph could no longer be seen when del Migliore wrote his description of it. Unfortunately, its absence was not due to its destruction during renovation but to the fact that it never existed, nor, for that matter, had Salvino degli Armati. It seems that del Migliore, an ardent Florentine patriot, had discovered and described a monument that no one had noted in the previous three centuries and that had conveniently been destroyed before he wrote about it. Both the discovery and the monument were products of del Migliore's patriotic imagination. If Redi could honor Pisa by claiming eyeglasses for a Pisan (Spina), del Migliore could make the same claim for a citizen of Florence, and even suggest in passing that Spina was also a Florentine, not a Pisan. And for many who followed, Salvino came to be accepted, especially in Florence, as the inventor of eyeglasses. In the nineteenth century, Libri, an eminent historian of mathematics and, of course, a Florentine by birth, revived this story. He was unhappy with his fellow citizens who had failed to honor a compatriot who had brought glory to their city by his notable invention, the importance of which the Florentines had neither understood nor appreciated. Libri noted that the original monument supposedly erected in 1317 no longer existed, and Florentines had to do something to honor Salvino degli Armati. In order to rectify their horrible and prolonged oversight, in 1841 the citizens of Florence placed an epitaph in the church of Santa Maria Maggiore. This nineteenth-century monument gave tangible support to a seven-teenth-century myth. It consisted of an epitaph that became coupled with an ancient marble bust. Together they remained on display for over half a century, in the cloister adjoining the church of Santa Maria Maggiore, as the official recognition of Salvino. In 1892 the cloister fell victim not to mere renovation but to urban renewal (or perhaps slum clearance). The structure was torn down to make way for a school. As was only proper, the school was named after Salvino himself. The ersatz monument was moved to a chapel in the interior of Santa Maria Maggiore, where it can still be seen today, although it is not one of the highlights of a trip to Florence. It probably deserves greater attention as one of the few memorials to a man who never existed. Nowhere in the records of Florence can the birth of Salvino degli Armati be verified, nor his life, nor his death. Yet he has a school named after him and an invention attributed to him, and, of course, an epitaph in a great church. How someone who was never born, never lived, and never died could have made a great contribution to mankind by inventing eyeglasses remains a mystery. Myths, it seems, especially patriotic ones, have lives of their own.

The only other candidate named for the title of inventor of eyeglasses is Roger Bacon (1214–1292). Roger Bacon, a member of the Franciscan order known to his successors as "doctor mirabilis," was born near Ilchester, England, where he received a master's degree. He then studied in Paris, where he received another master's degree and remained for several years to lecture on Aristotle and write on theology, mathematics, optics, and geography. His knowledge and expertise in optics are well documented and make him, in many ways, a more formidable candidate. After his return to England, his attacks on the Franciscans, Dominicans, and secular priests resulted in condemnation of his books and his imprisonment from 1277 to 1292. He died shortly after his release from prison.

Bacon has been proclaimed to be the inventor of the magnetic compass, gunpowder, and flying machines, and it has been said that he predicted the discovery of the New World. Most of these suggestions are, unfortunately, exaggerations. Gunpowder, for instance, was already in common use as a children's toy long before Bacon's alleged discovery of it.

The first suggestion that Bacon invented eyeglasses was made some 400 years after his death by the Anglo-Irish philosopher and scientist William Molyneux of Dublin. A careful reading of the Latin text of Bacon's writings does not support this interpretation. Although Bacon did write about the use of glass lenses to improve vision, the most that he can be credited with is the use of a magnifying glass. It is unfortunate, but true, that Bacon described only the use of a lens that was held close to the object, never one that was worn on the nose.

Like the Salvino hoax, the Bacon hypothesis had a nineteenth-century reincarnation. In 1845 F. E. de Caesemaker lent his name as author to a book written by Theodore Adrien Lievin Schellinck. This book claimed that Roger Bacon, living in Belgium at the time, gave an assortment of eyeglasses to Henry of Ghent, who on a trip to Italy showed them to Spina in Pisa. After all, Spina was not originally claimed as the inventor of eyeglasses, but was described in these words: "a monk of most excellent character and most acute mind, who understood everything that he heard said or saw done; and when it happened that somebody else was the first to invent eyeglasses and was unwilling to communicate the invention to others, all by himself he made them and goodnaturedly shared them with everybody." Thus it was all neatly tied together: from Bacon to Henry of Ghent to Spina to the world. Poor Salvino degli Armati played no role here.

Unlike Redi and del Migliore, who never even hinted that they might have stretched the truth, the actual author of this elaborate hoax confessed his misdeeds. Schellinck (1797–1867) was a poor and unscrupulous journalist, and in his autobiography he admitted that the Bacon hypothesis published over Caesemaker's name was a hoax that he had perpetrated after having received monetary support from some well-to-do Belgians, who apparently wished to honor their country by giving it a role in this great advance.

Despite four centuries of historical investigations, frauds, hoaxes, and mistakes, the inventor of eyeglasses remains anonymous. Neither a specific locale nor a specific man can be honored. Perhaps it has been more fun this way.

Addendum 1: The Death of Cleopatra

"It is a swamp adder!" cried Holmes—"the deadliest snake in India. He has died within ten seconds of being bitten. Violence does, in truth, recoil upon the violent, and the schemer falls into the pit which he digs for another."

A. Conan Doyle, *The Adventure of the Speckled Band*.

The circumstances surrounding the death of Cleopatra following the defeat of Mark Anthony by Augustus Caesar would seem to be a subject for historians to debate. However, the most thorough investigation of this matter was carried out by two physicians who would never have claimed that they were historians. The two physicians were Giovanni Battista Morgagni (1682–1771) and Giovanni Maria Lancisi (1655–1720). Morgagni is far better remembered today, and justly so, because he made a singular contribution to the history of medicine. Physicians before Morgagni often had progressed beyond the ancient humoral concepts of disease, and frequently they had localized diseases to specific regions, but they did not go much beyond this. They dealt in terms of diseases of the abdomen, diseases of the chest, diseases of the head. Morgagni went one critical step further and traced disorders to specific organs, such as the liver, lungs, heart. Later, Bichat began to trace diseases to specific tissues, and Virchow finally traced them to individual cells. But the critical leap from general region to specific organ was first made by Morgagni.

Morgagni was born in Forli and apparently was a precocious youth who wrote poetry and essays by the age of 11. He studied medicine at Bologna with Albertini, who first correlated dyspnea with heart disease, and with Valsalva, who described the anatomy of the ear, as well as the maneuver that still bears his name. While in Bologna, Morgagni assisted Valsalva in displaying anatomy to medical students, and he developed an interest in anatomy and pathology that lasted throughout his life. He published his first work in anatomy in 1706, and 5 years later he became professor of practical medicine at Padua. In 1715 he was given the chair of anatomy, the same chair that previously had belonged to Vesalius and Falloppio, among others. He held this position until his death in 1771, and during his six decades in the position he continually demonstrated his great talents as a scholar, teacher, physician, philosopher, pathologist, and medical historian. When he was 79 he published his most famous work, *De sedibus et causis morborum* (*The Seats and Causes of Disease*). This involved five books made up of some 70 letters that together constitute the foundation of modern pathologic anatomy, with an attempt being made to correlate clinical records with postmortem findings. In his preface, Morgagni modestly disavowed any special claim to originality and gave due credit to the works of his predecessors. It is true that many earlier authors had recorded the results of autopsy findings in an attempt to explain the cause of death. But in Morgagni's writings there is, for the first time, a vast array of pathologic findings that are well arranged and indexed. Each pathologic entity is presented after a detailed history of the patient's disease, including the symptoms and the treatment used; finally, a discussion of the relationship between the clinical picture and the autopsy findings concludes each study. Morgagni's knowledge of the literature of the subject is apparent throughout, as he discusses previous writings on each subject and meticulously gives each previous author full credit for his own observations. He often begins with ancient Greek sources and reviews the entire literature down to his own time.

The vast scope of his work and his numerous descriptions of "new" diseases made pathology a genuine branch of medicine. Morgagni gave the first description of (1) cerebral gummata due to syphilis, (2) diseases of the cardiac valves, such as aortic stenosis, pulmonary stenosis, and mitral insufficiency, (3) acute yellow atrophy of the liver, (4) tuberculosis of the kidney, (5) syphilitic aneurysm (although he did not know the cause), (6) meningitis secondary to acute otitis, (7) cancer of the stomach, (8) endocarditis, (9) coarctation of the aorta, (10) heart block (Stokes-Adams syndrome), which he described as "epilepsy with a slow pulse," (11) regional ileitis, (12) pneumonia with consolidation of the lung. Through his detailed clinical-anatomic studies he proved Valsalva's dictum that the cerebral insult in a stroke is on the cerebral hemisphere opposite to the side of the resulting paralysis. His work constituted a great stride toward the final cleansing of pathology of humoral concepts of disease.

Morgagni's approach is best grasped by reading his letters. It is hardly fair to let just one or two selections represent his contributions, but they can serve to give the flavor of his work. In Book II (Letter XXVI) he gave a description of cardiac failure due to mitral stenosis:

> Article 33: This old man was, to appearance, about sixty years of age, and had three months before been in the hospital, complaining of a difficulty of breathing, and spitting up an ill condition'd matter. Having been in the country lately, about the beginning of March, in the year 1742, and having been expos'd to a cold wind, upon his return home again, he was seiz'd in the night with a very great difficulty of breathing. Wherefore being brought into the same hospital again, in the morning, and sitting a little time by the fireside, while they were warming his bed, he had scarcely laid himself down therein, but he instantly died.
>
> The thorax, therefore, immediately cut into, and the sternum being taken away, the lungs appear'd to be so turgid as to fill up the whole cavities;.... There was, in both cavities of the thorax, a considerable quantity of water, not turbid, but the colour of urine; which kind of water, also, was found in the pericardium in somewhat larger quantities than it is generally.... The left ventricle ... seem'd to be wider than natural, and the mitral valves to be hard and thick; and all the semilunar valves had their edges hard, white, and what is more than all the rest, becomes so much thicken'd as to equal a line and a half of the inch of bologna in thickness.

In Book III (Letter XXXVII) Morgagni gave the history and findings in a case of acute yellow atrophy of the liver. This and many other cases in these books were based on cases of his old teacher Valsalva and were reported secondhand.

> Article 2: A young priest was seiz'd with the jaundice, a little after a kind of perturbation of mind: this disorder was also attended with a pain at the region of

the stomach, and a vomiting, by means of which he threw up both his food, and his medicines, frequently.... The physician did not observe any fever, till the close of the third day; at which time it discover'd itself with great violence, with a delirium, and convulsions of such a nature, that the patient was oblig'd to gnaw every thing with his teeth, and by his great strugglings almost overcame the strength of those who were about him; besides these, he was troubled with a vomiting of a darkish-coloured matter.... He died on the beginning of the fifth day.

The belly being open'd, the liver was found to be flaccid, and inclining to a palish colour; in the gall-bladder was a darkish bile.

Book I (Letter I) contains his description of a cerebral gumma in a young woman:

Being first affected with the lues venerea, and after that with a fever, join'd to severe pains of the head and delirium, she died of this complication of disorders in the hospital at Padua.... The dura mater, where it lay nearest the upper middle region of the lateral sinus on the right side, was much thicken'd and perfectly coalesc'd with the pia mater, and even with the substance of the brain: the meninges and brain were in part also semiputrid and glar'd with a very disagreeable colour, which was compos'd of a yellowish, mix'd with an ash like hue, especially in the cortical part of the cerebrum.

Morgagni was not merely a pathologist who spent his life dissecting bodies. He was a great humanist, a true scholar, a historian, a philosopher, and a renowned clinician and consultant. Nowhere is his broad, far-reaching humanism more apparent than in his letters to Lancisi.

Giovanni Maria Lancisi was born in Rome in 1654 and educated at the Collegio Romano and then at the University of Rome, from which he received his degree in medicine at the age of 18. He began his professional career as an assistant physician at the hospital of St. Spirito in Rome. In 1688, while prosector of anatomy at Collegio della Sapienza, he was called on to treat Pope Innocent XI for a renal stone. Following his successful treatment of this malady, he was appointed as official physician to the pope. He continued as official physician to the next two popes, Clement XI and Innocent XII. Lancisi was active as an anatomist, physiologist, botanist, pathologist, and clinician, but he is best remembered today as what we would call an epidemiologist. He described the epidemics of influenza in 1709–10, of cattle plague in 1713, and of malarial fever in 1715. His great treatise on swamp fevers (1717) shows clear insight into the theory of contagion and the possibility of transmission by mosquitoes. He also wrote an important book on the causes of sudden death, *De subitaneis mortis*, which was published in 1707. This was written because of the marked agitation of the Roman populace over the apparently large numbers of sudden deaths the previous year. This book, based on a number of personally conducted autopsies, describes cerebral hemorrhages and cardiac hypertrophy and dilatation as causes of sudden death. It also contains one of the first descriptions of vegetations of the heart valves. His later study on the heart and aneurysms, *De motu cordis et aneurysmatibus* (1728), which appeared after his death, is often described as a landmark in the history of cardiology (Fig. 1). In his discussion of the causes of cardiac enlargement, Lancisi mentioned heredity, insufficient or leaky valves, calcified valves and arteries, and conditions

JOANNIS MARIÆ

LANCISII

A Secretiori Cubiculo, & Archiatri Pontificii

DE MOTU CORDIS
ET
ANEURYSMATIBUS

OPVS POSTHVMVM

IN DUOS LIBROS DIVISUM.

EDITIO ROMANA SECUNDA

Quamplurimis acceſſionibus aucta.

ROMÆ MDCCXLV.

EX TYPOGRAPHIA PALLADIS

APUD FRATRES PALEARINOS.

SVPERIORVM FACVLTATE.

FIG. 1. Title page of Lancisi's *De Motu Cordis et Aneurysmatibus* (Courtesy of the Vatican Library.)

outside the heart, such as chronic asthma. In the section on aneurysms, he distinguished between true and false aneurysms and described aneurysms of syphilitic origin. Although Paré and Fernel had previously suggested that there was a relationship between syphilis and aneurysms, Lancisi was the first to make a definitive statement that syphilis was the cause of aneurysms of the aorta. In this book he also described the coronary circulation in detail and noted narrowing of the coronary blood vessels. Lancisi died in 1720 and left his entire fortune to the hospital of S. Spirito, to which he had previously given his large valuable library.

While Lancisi was his physician, Pope Clement XI charged him with the responsibility of resurrecting and publishing the copper anatomic plates of the great Bartolomeo Eustachio (1520–1574). Eustachio, whose name is associated with the tube he described connecting the ear and nasal pharynx, had completed these 47 plates in 1552, and they were believed to be even more accurate than those of Valsalva. The plates were finally published, with an introduction and commentary by Lancisi, in 1714. The pope was greatly pleased and asked Lancisi to see another unpublished work, *Methallotheca vaticana*, by Michele Mercati, through to publication. Under Lancisi's guidance and editorship, this was published in 1717, and it resulted in the "Cleopatra letters" between Lancisi and Morgagni.

One of the illustrations used by Lancisi to accompany Mercati's manuscript was an engraving by Maximilian Joseph Limpach, a Bohemian-born artist who lived and worked in Rome. This engraving, which was included in the book by order of Pope Clement XI, shows a marble statue of the dying Cleopatra with a snake wound around her arm. The text that accompanied this illustration raised the question whether Cleopatra had died as a result of being bitten by the snake or by drinking its poison. This engraving showed Cleopatra as a woman of great beauty, an opinion that contemporary coin portraits (Figs. 2 through 6) and even Plutarch's description do not support:

> *For her beauty . . . was in itself not altogether incomparable, nor such as to strike those who saw her; but converse with her had an irresistible charm, and her presence, combined with the persuasiveness of her discourse and the character which was somehow diffused about her behavior towards others, had something stimulating about it.*

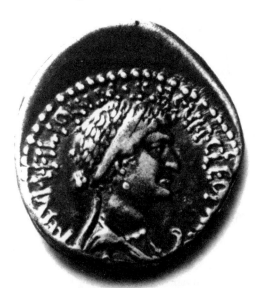

FIG. 2. Denarius of Mark Antony showing profile of Cleopatra (32 B.C.E.).

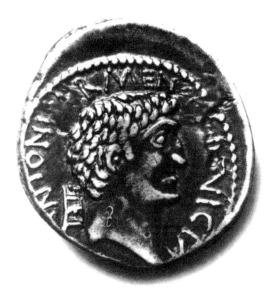

FIG. 3. Denarius of Mark Antony showing his profile (32 B.C.E.).

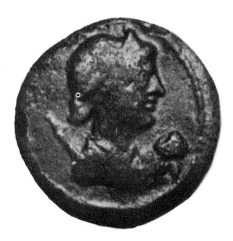

FIG. 4. Cleopatra as depicted on a contemporary bronze coin.

Plutarch, of course, was not a contemporary of Cleopatra. He was probably born during the reign of Claudius, about 45 or 50 C.E., in Boeotia, the area of Greece around Thebes. He studied in Athens and spent most of his life in Greece, where he set down his "parallel lives," a series of biographic sketches of Greeks and Romans. He described Cleopatra and her death in his "Life of Marc Antony":

> Some relate that an asp was brought in amongst those figs and covered with the leaves, and that Cleopatra had arranged that it might settle on her before she

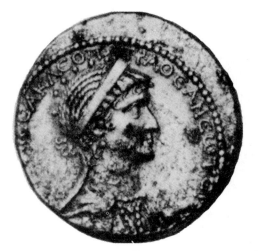

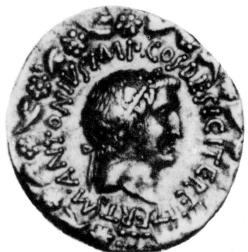

FIG. 5. Cleopatra (A) and Mark Antony (B) as shown on a cistophorus (30 B.C.E.).

knew, but, when she took away some of the figs and saw it, she said "So here it is," and held out her bare arm to be bitten. Others say that it was kept in a vase, and that she vexed and pricked it with a golden spindle till it seized her arm. But what really took place is known to no one, since it was also said that she carried poison in a hollow bodkin, about which she wound her hair; yet there was not so much as a spot found, or any symptom of poison upon her body, nor was the asp seen within the monument; only something like the trail of it was said to have been noticed on the sand by the sea, on the part towards which the building faced and where the windows were. Some relate that two faint puncture-marks were found on Cleopatra's arm, and so to this account Caesar seems to have given credit; for in his triumph there was carried a figure of Cleopatra, with an asp clinging to her. Such are the various accounts.

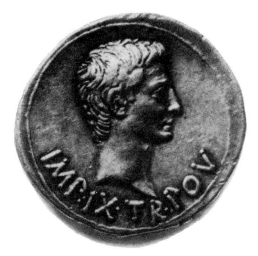

FIG. 6. Augustus Caesar as shown on a cistophorus (c. 20 B.C.E.).

Morgagni, after seeing the engraving of the dying Cleopatra, wrote to Lancisi to pursue the issue of the cause of Cleopatra's death. The ensuing correspondence was not a succession of dull scientific documents exchanged by two forensic pathologists but a series of erudite missives that demonstrate the breadth of learning of these two great physicians and humanists. Morgagni noted that the engraving showed Cleopatra dying with an asp attached to her arm. But did this mean that she died of the bite of the asp or that the asp was there merely to show that snake venom, however taken, was the cause of her death? He then reviewed the data:

1. Propertius, who described the statues of Cleopatra that were carried in the triumphal procession of Augustus, noted that the statues were covered with numerous asps.

2. Florus wrote that Cleopatra applied snakes to her veins and was freed by death, as if in sleep.

3. Dio doubted the snakebite theory.

4. Horace confirmed that she was bitten by an asp:

> Yet she, seeking to die a nobler death, showed for the dagger's point no woman's fear, nor sought to win with her swift fleet some secret shore; she even dared to gaze with face serene upon her fallen palace; courageous too, to handle poisonous asps, that she might draw black venom to her heart, waxing bolder as she resolved to die.

Morgagni himself was able to find no ancient descriptions of Cleopatra having drunk snake venom. In fact, he related that Celsus taught that snake venom kills only when injected into a wound, not when swallowed.

Lancisi accepted the challenge. He refused to accept the testimony of Horace, who was not present at Cleopatra's death and who as a poet may not have respected truth as much as beauty. He believed that there was no definite proof that Cleopatra died of a snakebite, and his belief was that she died from taking some readily available form of poison. The debate continued for two more letters, with these two adversaries tossing back and forth the opinions of Plutarch, Dio, Florus, Suetonius, Horace, Propertius, and Redi—our old friend Francesco Redi, who, imbued with the spirit of Galileo, attempted to answer such questions with experimental data. Redi had worked directly with vipers to learn whether or not their poisons were effective when swallowed, whether or not an asp expels all its venom with a single bite, and whether or not a single asp could have bitten Cleopatra and her two handmaidens. Fortunately for us, Redi's data were not conclusive, for occasionally he noted that all of the venom was not expelled until the fifth or sixth bite. Because nothing ends arguments as decisively as data, it is fortunate that Redi's study, although it confirmed Celsus's opinion and ruled out the drinking of venom, did not rule out the one-asp hypothesis and thus allowed Morgagni and Lancisi to tax their knowledge of ancient authors and explore the cause of Cleopatra's death.

Addendum 2: Botticelli's Sign

> Botticelli, one of the greatest painters of the Italian Renaissance, demonstrated the Babinski reflex more than 400 years before the publication of Babinski's first description of this reflex.
>
> T. E. Cone and S. Koshbin (1978)

The overlap between science and the humanities in Renaissance Florence that was typified by the poetry of Redi and the broad range of historical learning of Morgagni and Lancisi was not limited to physicians and their contributions to art and literature. Artists also contributed to medicine. The anatomic studies of DaVinci serve as a constant reminder of this. More recently, Cone and Koshbin (*American Journal of Diseases of Children* 132:188, 1978) have suggested that at least one artist, Sandro Botticelli (1445–1510), made a remarkable but long-ignored contribution to neurology by demonstrating the Babinski sign more than 400 years before Babinski did. In Botticelli's *Madonna and Child with Angels*, the Madonna is shown holding the infant Jesus and stroking his foot. Dorsiflexion of the great toe of this foot is also shown, and to these authors this suggested that such dorsiflexion was

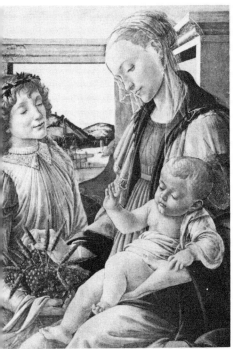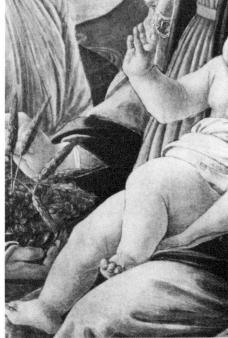

FIG. 7. Left: *The Madonna of the Eucharist* from the Isabella Steward Gardner Museum. **Right:** Detail of *The Madonna of the Eucharist* showing dorsiflexion of right great toe and peculiar hand posturing.

235

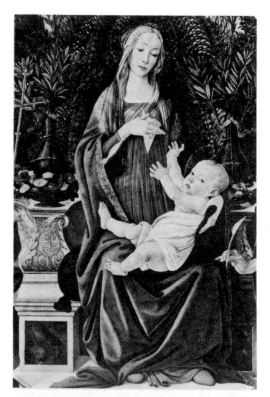

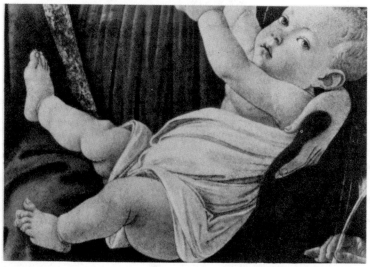

FIG. 8. **Above:** Detail from *Virgin and Child with the Two Saints John*, painted in 1485, from the Berlin Museum. Note stylized postures of hands, as well as dorsiflexion of great toe. **Below:** Closer detail.

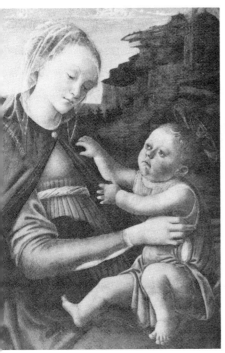
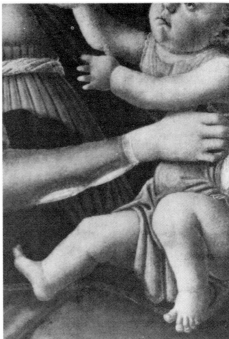

FIG. 9. Left: Detail from *Madonna Guidi*, from the Louvre. Note dorsiflexion of great toes.
Right: Closer detail.

known to Botticelli to be a normal response of a normal infant to such stimulation. The implications of this hypothesis are profound. Even Babinski did not know that this was a normal phenomenon among children during early life until he had been studying the response for several years. Botticelli must have been both thorough and perceptive to have noted this response of infants to a strong, usually noxious stimulus. Unfortunately, a more thorough review of Botticelli's works cannot support this hypothesis. It is true that Botticelli, as a student of Fra Filippo Lippi, had learned the importance of studying live infants in order to more accurately portray the newborn Jesus. In his work, the proportions of the infant do reflect those of a real infant rather than those of a miniaturized adult. But a survey of his other paintings shows numerous examples of infants with dorsiflexed great toes without the benefit of any stimulation of the sole of the foot. (Figs. 7 through 12). This suggests that Botticelli did not see any causal physiological relationship between stimulation of the sole of the foot and a resulting dorsiflexion of the great toe. Close observation and physiological reasoning cannot be the basis of this arrangement of anatomy. Some other explanation must be sought, and it can be found in Botticelli's art itself, which is replete with stylistic mannerisms, the symbolism of which may or may not be apparent to us. These include formalized postures of the arms, hands, fingers, and, it would seem, toes. Overall, "Botticelli's sign" seems to be one of his numerous stylistic mannerisms or symbols, not a result of perceptive physiological observations.

The only available discussion of the Morgagni-Lancisi correspondence is a delightful article by Saul Jarcho ("The Correspondence of Morgagni and Lancisi on the Death of Cleopatra," *Bulletin of the History of Medicine* 43:299–325, 1969). This, like so many of Jarcho's articles, instructs us in facets of medicine long ignored or overlooked. Morgagni's *The Seats and Causes of Disease, Investigated by Anatomy* was translated into English by Bengamin Alexander in 1769. This has recently been beautifully reprinted by Hafner Publishing Company. Morgagni's life and work have been discussed by Saul Jarcho ("Giovanni Battista Morgagni: His Interests, Ideas and Achievements," *Bulletin of the History of Medicine* 22:503–527, 1948), and Lancisi's life has been recorded by J. Foot (*International Clinic* 2:292–308, 1917). Lester King's *The Medical World of the Eighteenth Century* (University of Chicago Press, 1958) remains the best overview of medicine at the time of Morgagni and Lancisi.

NOTES

Anyone interested in pursuing a more detailed investigation of the invention of eyeglasses is advised to avoid all standard histories of medicine and instead search out the writings of Edward Rosen, especially the following:

1. Rosen, E. (1956): The invention of eyeglasses, Part I. *J. Hist. Med.*, 13:13–46.

2. Rosen, E. (1956): The invention of eyeglasses, Part II. *J. Hist. Med.*, 13:183–218.

3. Rosen, E. (1953): Carlo Dation the inventor of eyeglasses. *Isis*, 44:4–10.

4. Rosen, E. (1954): Did Roger Bacon invent eyeglasses? *Arch. Int. of Hist. of Science*, 7:3–15.

These four articles have been the main source for the history as given here.

The best available biography of Redi is by Rufus Cole (*Annals of Medical History* 8:349–360, 1926).